VGM Opportunities Series

OPPORTUNITIES IN
PHYSICIAN CAREERS

Jan Sugar-Webb

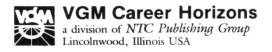

VGM Career Horizons
a division of *NTC Publishing Group*
Lincolnwood, Illinois USA

ABF 4865

Cover Photo Credits:
Front cover: upper left and upper right,
Columbus-Cabrini Medical Center photos;
lower left, NTC photo; lower right, George
Washington University Medical Center photo.
Back cover: upper left, upper right, and
lower left, Columbus-Cabrini Medical Center
photos; lower right, LaGrange Memorial
Hospital photo.

Library of Congress Cataloging-in-Publication Data

Sugar-Webb, Jan, 1954–
    Opportunities in physician careers / Jan Sugar-Webb.

        p.   cm. — (VGM opportunities series)
    ISBN 0-8442-8595-1 (hardbound): $12.95. — ISBN 0-8442-8597-8
(softbound): $9.95
    1. Medicine—Specialties and specialists. 2. Medicine—Vocational
guidance. I. Title. II. Series.
    [DNLM: 1. Career Choice. 2. Specialties, Medical. W 21 S947o]
R729.5.S6S84   1990
610'.69—dc20
DNLM/DLC
for Library of Congress   90-12879
                                                                      CIP

1996 Printing

Published by VGM Career Horizons, a division of NTC Publishing Group.
©1991 by NTC Publishing Group, 4255 West Touhy Avenue,
Lincolnwood (Chicago), Illinois 60646-1975 U.S.A.
Manufactured in the United States of America.
        6 7 8 9 VP 9 8 7 6 5 4 3

ABOUT THE AUTHOR

Jan Sugar-Webb, M.A., is an award-winning communications and marketing consultant in Chicago. Through her communications firm, Sugar Webb & Associates, she frequently works with health care organizations and physicians. She is a former director of public affairs at Mount Sinai Hospital on Chicago's West Side. Prior to that appointment, she was a research and policy writer for the American Medical Association, where she worked on the "Health Policy Agenda for the American People," the AMA's blueprint for the delivery of health care in the twenty-first century.

Ms. Sugar-Webb holds a B.A. degree in literature from Simmons College in Boston and a master's degree in education from Boston University. Her broad experience as a teacher includes directing a program for high school dropouts from the inner city and implementing a training program for teachers of the disabled at City Colleges of Chicago.

FOREWORD

Medicine is a unique profession. Few careers offer the excitement, challenge, and rewards available to the talented physician. And never in its long history has medicine been as complex as it is today. Students contemplating a medical career face a multitude of choices before they ever take the Hippocratic oath. Medical students must decide to pursue one of dozens of medical specialties and subspecialties. They may find their niche in the operating room or a research lab, in a city or a small town, working with elderly patients or infants. *Opportunities in Physician Careers* provides a way for students to begin to explore these options.

As medicine evolves, the education and preparation of physicians also changes. Beginning in 1991, the Medical College Admission Test (MCAT) will be substantially different than in the past. The long hours sometimes worked by residents have become more controversial and are also being reevaluated in the continuing effort to educate qualified physicians.

The results of these educational efforts are of crucial importance to all Americans. As we face the AIDS crisis and struggle to meet the health care needs of an increasingly older population, the need for qualified physicians is constant. More and more students are deciding to meet that need. The opportunities are there for all, and the number of women and minorities entering medical schools is increasing.

For those who decide to become physicians, the career demands long hours and personal sacrifices. It also offers great financial and personal rewards—including the respect of society and the satisfaction of preserving and improving the lives of others.

The Editors
VGM Career Books

CONTENTS

CHAPTER 1

PHYSICIANS—YESTERDAY AND TODAY

> Where there is love for humanity, there also is love for
> the art of medicine.
>> Hippocrates

Hippocrates is the father of modern medicine. He gave medicine a scientific basis and moral inspiration that it lacked before. Yet, the practice of medicine in various forms existed before Hippocrates developed his system of observation—it is as old as humankind. Human beings have always shared with other animals the need to protect and care for themselves.

PRIMITIVE MEDICINE

Primitive medicine was steeped in the belief that spirits were the cause of death and disease. A spirit caused disease by invading the body and producing pain or by withdrawing vitality, causing the life force to wane. But medicine was only one part of a larger belief system which held that a whole set of mystical processes was responsible for natural occurrences. Rain, fire, fertility, and crop growth were all controlled by unseen spirits. Therefore, the first physician was a sorcerer of sorts, a person who promoted well-being by warding off evil spirits.

A cave in France, known as the Cave of the Three Brothers, houses what is likely the oldest picture of a healer. In the painting, done on a wall in the cave perhaps 25,000 years ago, the figure is dancing; he has human feet but the paws of a bear. Antlers sprout out of his head. His eyes stare outward. This person, it seems, is a tribal doctor, wrapped in animal skins, driving evil spirits away. His ability to do magic is inseparable from his ability to heal the sick.

ANCIENT EGYPTIANS

Archaeological evidence abounds to demonstrate the existence of disease and interventions such as herb therapies and surgery. But, the oldest historic phase of medicine known is that of ancient Egypt.

Ancient Egyptians believed in immortality, that the soul would return to the body sometime after death. Egyptians preserved the bodies of the dead along with treasured possessions. They documented events on writing material called papyrus. It is from preserved medical papyri that our knowledge of ancient Egyptian medicine is derived.

The most famous medical papyri, and those which contain the most information, are named after the men who obtained them in Egypt and shared them with the world—Smith and Ebers. The Smith papyrus essentially outlines 48 surgical cases, including diagnosis and method of treatment. It deals exclusively with wounds and fractures. The suggested treatment for the cases is mostly practical, but includes a mix of magical incantations against pestilence and a few magical remedies, including one ''to change an old man into a youth of twenty.'' Medicine had not gained its own status at the beginning of documented Egyptian medicine; it still involved magic.

Notwithstanding, the Smith papyrus is an impressive document. The author of the original papyrus was probably a gifted surgeon who used practical interventions, like the following recommendation for treating a fractured collarbone:

> You must lay him down outstretched on his back, with something folded between his two shoulder blades. Then you must spread his two shoulder blades so that his two collarbones stretch, so that the fracture falls into its proper place. Then you must make him two compresses of cloth. Then you must place one of them inside his upper arm, the other below his upper arm...

Sometimes the treatments recommended are still used today. When the ailing patient has a dislocated jaw, the doctor is instructed to put his or her thumbs inside the patient's mouth. The doctor's other fingers go under the patient's chin, and the doctor guides the jaw back into its proper place. This treatment is still the only treatment used for a dislocated jaw. The Smith papyrus contains graphic information about more serious injuries as well.

The Ebers papyrus, which was probably composed around 2000 B.C., contains some surgical material, but is mostly a text on internal medicine. It names diseases and remedies as well as some cosmetic aids. The prescriptions in this papyrus include not only the names of remedies, but amounts to take as well. Like the Smith papyrus, parts of the Ebers papyrus contain observant medical data:

> If you examine a person who suffers from pains in the stomach and is sick in the arm, the breast, and the stomach, and it appears that it is the disease uat, you will say: 'Death has entered into the mouth and has taken its seat there.' You will prepare a remedy composed of the following plants: the stalks of the plant tehus, mint, the red seeds of the plant sechet; and you will have them cooked in beer; you will give it to the sick person and his arm will be easily extended without pain, and then you will say, 'The disease has gone out from the intestine through the anus, it is not necessary to repeat the medicine.'

The Ebers papyrus also contains more magical treatments for diseases, like a frog warmed in oil for a burn. (This treatment is to be accompanied by a chant.) Nevertheless, the Greeks acknowledge the Egyptians' groundwork in the areas of surgery and medical intervention.

Although contributions to medicine came from many eras in history and many places in the world, there is none that has had as pervasive an influence on modern Western medicine as the contribution made by the Greeks. Nowhere in Homer's *Iliad,* written between 900 and 800 B.C., does he mention any incantations to treat the wounds of war. Homer writes of treatments that were strictly medical.

HIPPOCRATES AND THE INFLUENCE OF GREEK MEDICINE

The most famous of the Greek physicians was Hippocrates, born around 460 B.C. He is credited with the development of the scientific method which included careful, detailed observation of the patient. Hippocrates wrote:

> In acute diseases the physician must make his observations in the following way. He must first look at the face of the patient and see whether it is like that of people in good health, and, particularly, whether it is like its usual self, for this is the best of all; whereas the most opposite to it is the worst, such as the following; nose sharp, eyes hollow, temples sunken, ears cold and contracted and their lobes turned out, and the skin about the face dry, tense, and parched, the color of the face as a whole being yellow or black, livid or lead colored...

Hippocrates also taught that wounds should be washed in boiled water and that doctors' hands should be clean. Many of the observations that he and his pupils made about the human body are still valid in terms of modern Western medicine. He wrote:

> When sleep puts an end to delirium it is a good sign.
> Weariness without cause indicates disease.
> If there be a painful affection in any part of the body,
>   but no suffering, there is mental disorder.

Because of Hippocrates' moral idea of what a physician should be—a professional assisting in the healing process in every way—graduating medical students today take the Hippocratic oath.

Hippocratic medicine was continued later in the Egyptian medical school founded by two Greeks, Herophilus and Erasistratus. They dissected human bodies and learned about how the organs worked. Roman medicine was also developed by Greeks. The Greek physician Galen, who was born in A.D. 130, studied anatomy and physiology. For over a thousand years after he died, his writings were considered to be the medical authority.

THE RENAISSANCE

Around A.D. 400 the dissolution of the Roman Empire resulted in a halt to the development of modern Western medicine for several centuries. After the eighth century, when the Arabs spread their empire from the Middle East to Spain, medical schools and hospitals began to flourish.

Several centuries later, the Renaissance was beginning, and new interest was aroused in medicine. During the fifteenth century, the Renaissance was at its pinnacle, and medicine was even advanced by artists like Leonardo Da Vinci who made careful drawings of the structure of the human body. Andreas Vesalius's book, *Fabric of the Human Body,* was published in 1543, and it advanced surgery throughout the world because it was the first real written anatomy of the human body.

THE SEVENTEENTH CENTURY— THREE CONTRIBUTIONS

During the seventeenth century, three major contributions to medicine were made. William Harvey, an English physician, wrote *De Motu Cordis et Sanguinis in Animalibus,* published in 1628. In it he describes his discovery of how blood circulates in the body. It has remained one of the most famous medical texts ever written both because of its enthusiastic style and because it outlines one of the most important medical discoveries ever made.

Later in the century, an Italian physiologist named Marcello Marpighi filled the gap left in Harvey's discoveries by creating the first description of the capillaries that connect arteries and veins.

The Dutch scientist Anthony van Leeuwenhoek refined the microscope. He used home-ground lenses with short focal lengths to observe what could not be seen before: red corpuscles, spermatozoa, and bacteria are a few examples.

THE EIGHTEENTH CENTURY—
THE BEGINNING OF PREVENTION

By the eighteenth century, much was known about the workings of the human body. Yet, the century had few original thinkers. Mostly it was a time of systematization and classification. Carl von Linné (or Linnaeus), the Swedish botanist and physician, established the idea of classification both in botany and in medicine. He was the originator of the binomial nomenclature in science classifying each natural object by a family name and a specific name, like homo sapiens for humans.

The few who made discoveries in the eighteenth century began to use medicine to prevent ill health. Sanitation improved; sewers were covered, and streets were paved. And, in 1796, Edward Jenner developed the first vaccine against smallpox. For years, smallpox epidemics killed many. When the smallpox vaccine was given to 12,000 people in London, the yearly rate of the disease dropped from 2,018 to 622.

Other important medical advances were made by Caspar Wolff and John Hunter. Caspar Friedrich Wolff, a German, is noted for his major contribution to modern embryology. Wolff noted that the embryo was not preformed and encased in the ovary, as previously believed, but rather that organs are formed "in leaf-like layers." John Hunter, a Scottish surgeon who practiced in London, was an influential physician and teacher who helped win respect for surgery as a scientific profession.

THE NINETEENTH CENTURY—
DIAGNOSIS AND BETTER TREATMENT

Modern medicine, as we would recognize it, began during the nineteenth century. The causes and treatments of many diseases were beginning to be understood. The nineteenth century also brought advances in medical research and the birth of modern surgery.

One key discovery occurred when a French physician, Jean Corvisart des Marets, found that certain parts of the body give different sounds when thumped. The sound changes if fluid is present. This important diagnostic tool is called percussing.

Another French physician, Réné-Théophile-Hyacinthe Laennec, invented the stethoscope in 1819. It is said that he found percussing the chest of one of his patients too difficult, and he rolled up a cylinder of paper in his hands and placed it against the patient's chest to listen. His publication of successive editions of *Traité de l'auscultation médiate* became the foundation of modern knowledge of diseases of the chest and their diagnosis.

Modern surgery was born in 1846 at Massachusetts General Hospital in Boston when William Morton first anesthetized a patient with ether. However, patients continued to die on the operating table from infection until the chemist Louis Pasteur's discovery that bacteria caused disease was taken seriously.

The Scottish surgeon, Joseph Lister, understood the importance of Pasteur's discovery. To implement this knowledge, he first tried to kill bacteria that entered his patients during surgery. Later, he tried to prevent bacteria from entering wounds by boiling instruments and using antiseptic solutions. Also using Pasteur's work, a German physician called Robert Koch experimented with his bacteria. He found the germ that causes tuberculosis and developed the science of bacteriology.

As the causes of disease were becoming more familiar, research began to flourish in the prevention of disease. The Russian bacteriologist Elie Metchnikoff discovered that certain white blood cells attack bacteria and other particles that enter the blood. And in 1890, a German surgeon discovered a cure for diphtheria. Karl Landsteiner discovered the four main blood types and made blood transfusion possible for the first time. And Paul Ehrlich, a German bacteriologist, invented a chemical compound that cured syphilis.

THE TWENTIETH CENTURY— REVOLUTIONARY PROGRESS

Medicine in the twentieth century is a product of all the observation and discovery that came before it. The remarkable progress of the twentieth century falls mostly under the category of prevention. Medicine in the twentieth century has concentrated on the prevention of occurrence, recurrence, and spread of diseases. Understanding of the human body is very sophisticated in the twentieth century. Many tools for diagnosis have become available, making experimentation much more possible than ever before. Wilhelm Röentgen first developed X-rays in 1895, but started applying them to medical use in the early 1900s. Röentgen's discovery gave diagnostic medicine its sure footing and immeasurably advanced surgery as a science.

England made a major contribution to medicine in 1928, when Sir Alexander Fleming made the chance observation that staphylococcus actually dissolved when *Penicillium notatum* contaminated the culture. He extracted an active principle that he called penicillin and found it to be superior in treating infection. More work was done later that led to the mass production of penicillin in the late 1940s.

After World War II, there was a vast increase in medical research. The United States government began to make a major contribution to research through the National Institutes of Health. In 1952 Jonas Salk first inoculated thirty disabled children in Pennsylvania to see if his vaccine would raise antibody levels. By 1955, after research and field trials, the Salk vaccine against polio was declared a success.

MEDICINE TODAY

Advances in therapeutics—diagnosis and drugs, surgery, diet, and sanitation—have helped to increase life span. Where once people died of polio, diphtheria, or smallpox, modern therapeutics have managed to either eliminate or treat formerly fatal diseases. Degenerative diseases have replaced many fatal diseases as the types of complaints often seen by modern practitioners. Modern life-styles and increased life span have resulted in a high incidence of cancer and heart disease, now managed by practitioners who specialize in these diseases.

The advent of medical research and the lengthening of life expectancy have contributed to the phenomenon of medical specialization. There are currently 23 medical specialty boards that accredit physicians and surgeons in those specialties. There are many more related subspecialties. Specialists concentrate on one part of the body, a specific age group, or on techniques developed to treat or diagnose certain disorders. Diagnostic procedures are so sophisticated today that there are some subspecialists who concentrate strictly on specific procedures.

The physician of tomorrow surely faces a more complicated decision than the physician of yesterday. Beginning in medical school, students are encouraged to investigate which part of medicine they will pursue. Medicine today isn't only clinical practice or research or teaching. It is all of those.

From specialty to specialty, there are many variables. Length of training, annual income, amount of contact with patients—all are factors that medical students must consider when choosing what type of physician they will become.

CHAPTER 2

EDUCATION AND PREPARATION

Medical education in America was not always the complicated process that it is today. One hundred years ago, medical school lasted less than a year, and the M.D. degree was granted regardless of grades. The minimum age requirement for being a doctor was 21, but it was a rule to which no one strictly adhered. Teaching was all done by lecture, and M.D.'s did not get clinical or research experience before beginning to practice. Medical schools were called proprietary schools because the lecturers who taught there (usually fewer than a dozen) often owned the schools.

In the mid-nineteenth century, events began to take place that were to change the face of American medical education. American doctors began to travel to Europe to learn the new laboratory methods that European doctors were using. At the same time, the modern university was emerging, and new regulatory authority was being assumed by state and federal governments. By 1910, when Abraham Flexner published his famous report which outlined the conditions in American and Canadian medical schools, the foundation for change was well underway.

As the body of medical knowledge grew, research and teaching were able to become full-time activities. By the late nineteenth century, the academic physician was very prominent. Today, the division between academic and clinical medicine still exists. And the development of the medical scholar has had an enduring impact on the way medical schools now operate.

GETTING INTO MEDICAL SCHOOL

There are 17,000 positions available yearly at the 127 medical schools in the United States. In the late 1980s, approximately 30,000 students competed for those places. These days, if you want to be a doctor, your chances are just over 50 percent of being accepted to medical school.

This chapter outlines the medical school entrance procedure and discusses the variables that help you gain entrance to medical school.

During High School

Some people already know when they're very young that they want to be doctors. There are several things that a high school student can do to prepare for medical school.

In order to see if you like or can handle the rigorous premedical courses necessary to get into medical school, you might try taking a few difficult science courses while still in high school.

Of equal importance is finding work that is related to the medical field. Whether you find a paid job in a lab during the summer or a volunteer position working in a hospice, you can learn a lot by being involved in the medical field before college. And a history of medically related jobs can be a powerful statement to an admissions committee.

Good grades and good study habits are important elements for preparing for a future in medicine. Medical school is a long and arduous process that takes more hard work and hours than perhaps any other profession. Early training in intense studying is an asset.

If you are sure while you are still in high school that you want to go to medical school, combined undergraduate and medical studies programs do exist. Many of the programs are six years long. Others take seven and eight years to complete. The programs avoid the medical school application process and let students take courses they would naturally pick without the constant worry about getting into medical school. The list of universities and colleges that have combined programs is found in Appendix D at the back of the book. It lists both accelerated and non-accelerated programs.

Grades in College

Medical school admission requirements vary as far as grades are concerned. Some medical schools don't even have a minimum grade point average requirement. You are a lot more assured of getting into a medical school, though, if you have at least a 3.0 grade point average.

Medical College Admissions Test

The Medical College Admissions Test (MCAT) is a strong determinant of medical school admission. The test usually takes just under ten hours to complete. The MCAT has been given by the Association of American Medical Colleges (AAMC) since 1930. As of 1977, the MCAT has consisted of four sections that are scored in six categories. Changes in medical education and medical practice have prompted the Association of American Medical Colleges to make extensive revisions in the MCAT. Beginning in the spring of 1991, the MCAT will be substantially different. Those applying for admission to medical school in 1992 will take the new MCAT.

The four new sections and the amount of time they will take will be as follows:

Verbal Reasoning	85 minutes
Physical Sciences	100 minutes
Writing Sample	60 minutes
Biological Sciences	100 minutes

The changes for the new revised MCAT will cut the current test time by at least 80 minutes.

MCAT review books are available as are professional review courses to help prepare people for the test. One text dealing with medical school admissions suggests nine months of preparation in order to obtain a high MCAT score. A new MCAT student manual will be in college bookstores in September 1990.

Coursework During College

Educational philosophies vary from school to school, but all medical schools agree on the benefits of a broad education. This means a strong foundation in the sciences as well as excellent communications skills and a background in the humanities.

General requirements for medical school are one year of biology, two years of chemistry (through organic chemistry), and one year of physics. The courses should be demanding and include adequate laboratory experience.

Many medical schools require or strongly recommend math courses. Math is useful in understanding chemistry, physics, biology, and also computers, which are in wide use at medical schools today.

A major in science is not necessary for medical school acceptance. In fact, in the 1989–1990 entering class, students who majored in the humanities had some of the highest acceptance rates. Students in economics, anthropology, English, and political science fared better that year than those majoring in chemistry, biochemistry, biology, and physiology.

Applying to Medical School

The application process to medical school is fraught with hope and fear for most students. Since gaining entrance is a combination of good grades and MCAT scores, recommendations, extracurricular activities, and your personal essay, it is no wonder that the process is a dizzying experience. There are so many variables that you can never be sure of the outcome.

The value of good grades and MCAT scores was mentioned earlier in the chapter. The following is a brief explanation of the other parts of the process leading to being granted an interview.

RECOMMENDATIONS

Typically, recommendations for medical school are letters written by people with whom you've had an academic or professional relationship during college. Professors and physicians with whom you've worked on medically related jobs are good candidates for letters of recommendation. An emerging trend in letters of recommendation is the composite recommendation. In this case, a premedical committee drafts a letter of recommendation using the letters of people you have chosen to recommend you.

EXTRACURRICULAR ACTIVITIES

Working in a hospital, clinic, or research facility will help you decide whether you want to be a physician. It also lets admissions committees know that you were motivated to answer that question, or that your activities in a medically related job propelled you into medicine.

If admissions committees only see applications that reflect grades and MCAT scores, they cannot see you as a whole person. Medical schools are looking for indicators that medicine is important to you for the right reasons and that you are a caring and humane individual.

Additionally, everyone likes people who are interesting. Don't hide the fact that you were an Outward Bound counselor, teach in an adult literacy program, or paint houses in the summers to pay for college.

THE ESSAY

The medical school essay is a way to get to know someone more personally before an interview. It is an opportunity for you to become more than a jumble of statistics on a sheet of paper. A well-written essay can go far in making people interested in you among all the other candidates. This is the place to tell the committee what is special about you and your reason for wanting to become a doctor.

According to the Gourman Report, published in 1989, the ten most competitive medical schools in alphabetical order are:

Columbia University, College of Physicians and Surgeons
Cornell University Medical College
Harvard Medical School
Johns Hopkins University School of Medicine
Stanford University School of Medicine
University of California, San Francisco
University of Chicago, Pritzker School of Medicine
University of Michigan Medical School
University of Pennsylvania School of Medicine
Yale University School of Medicine

MEDICAL SCHOOL TODAY

Medical education today is undergoing many changes. The 1980s brought an era of tightened fiscal management, as well as a questioning of medical school curriculum and residency training. In 1984, "The Report of the General Professional Education of the Physician" (GPEP) was published. GPEP made many recommendations for change in medical school curriculum. The 1990s is seeing a reappraisal of the medical education system.

Underrepresented Groups

One change in medical education has been in the composition of the student population at medical schools and, thus, eventually, in the physician population. Women now comprise 40 percent of medical school applicants, up from

8 percent fifteen years ago. The Association of American Medical Colleges (AAMC) estimates a 12 percent increase this year in female applicants compared with only a 3 percent rise in male applicants. (Men and women have similar acceptance and completion rates.) The percentage of women in the U.S. physician population has grown to almost 17 percent; in 1970 it was under 8 percent. Predictions are that by the year 2010 women will represent almost one-third of all physicians in the United States.

Although continuing efforts are made by medical schools and universities, some minorities are still underrepresented in medicine. Although black Americans represent approximately 12 percent of the U.S. population, they represented just over 6 percent of the first year medical students in 1989. Only 8 percent of all applicants to medical school were black in 1989, and 50 percent of black applicants were accepted.

Hispanics represent approximately 7 percent of the U.S. population, but only 4 percent of the total medical students. Native Americans represent 0.6 percent of the U.S. population, but only 0.4 percent of the medical school population.

The Curriculum

During the first several years, students receive instruction in anatomy, physiology, biochemistry, microbiology, pharmacology, pathology, and behavioral sciences. In some medical schools, students are introduced to interviewing and examining patients by the end of the first year. But whether patient contact is introduced in the first year or the second, almost all medical schools introduce clinical problems early in the curriculum.

Since GPEP, many schools have switched emphasis from discipline-based to problem-based learning. Problem-based learning is an instructional format that emphasizes small-group teaching, self-study, and a faculty member as facilitator of this learning process.

The third and fourth years of medical school are mainly devoted to clinical clerkships. The purpose of these clerkships is to prepare students for the patient-physician relationship, teach them to recognize basic disease patterns, and familiarize students with the specialties to enable them to choose a residency program.

CHAPTER 3

RESIDENCY TRAINING

After graduation from medical school, where the M.D. degree is conferred, physicians wanting to practice medicine go into a residency program in the area of medicine that interests them. These programs expand upon the knowledge and skills that medical schools offer, and provide residents with increased responsibility for patients in supervised settings. As discussed in chapter 1, health care has broadened its scope dramatically since World War II. In addition to other effects, the way physicians are trained has changed dramatically, too.

Fewer than 600 hospitals provided residency training for 5,000 physicians in 1940; in 1987, 1,558 institutions provided training for over 81,000 physicians. In addition to their basic goal of providing the physician with clinical skills, residency training also provides the opportunity for involvement in research, for applying technology to patient problems, and for becoming a part of the teaching of medical students, residents in earlier years of training, and other health professionals. The resident's unique position is that he or she provides service to patients while remaining a student of the residency program.

INTERNS, RESIDENTS, AND FELLOWS

The words internship, residency, and fellowship create some confusion when one is trying to understand training after medical school. Medical organizations, such as the American Medical Association (AMA), and hospitals call training after medical school graduate medical education (GME). Sometimes in hospitals the term housestaff is used. Housestaff refers to anyone participating in a hospital-based residency program.

The word internship has been used historically to mean anyone in the first year of training after medical school. In 1975, this first year of graduate medical education was integrated into the rest of residency training. The year that was formerly called internship is now called the first year of residency, or PGY-1, which stands for postgraduate year one. The word internship is still used in places.

Fellowship is used to mean subspecialty training after residency. For example, when physicians do three years of internal medicine training they are called residents during that training period. After that, if they want to specialize in cardiology, which is a subspecialty of internal medicine, they may go into a cardiology training program for three years and be called cardiology fellows. The definition of the word fellowship varies among the different specialty boards, specialty programs, and institutions. In some places, physicians in subspecialty training are simply called residents. For the purpose of this text, the word resident will be used to mean anyone participating in graduate medical education, whether it is specialty or subspecialty training. The words intern and fellow will not be used.

SPECIALIZATION

There are 24 approved medical specialties. They are governed by 23 medical specialty boards. The following is a list of these specialties:

Allergy and Immunology
Anesthesiology
Colon and Rectal Surgery
Dermatology
Emergency Medicine
Family Practice
Internal Medicine
Neurological Surgery
Neurology
Nuclear Medicine
Obstetrics and Gynecology
Ophthalmology
Orthopedic Surgery

Otolaryngology
Pathology
Pediatrics
Physical Medicine and Rehabilitation
Plastic Surgery
Preventive Medicine
Psychiatry
Radiology
Surgery
Thoracic Surgery
Urology

Along with these specialties are subspecialties. A subspecialist is someone who has completed specialty training and gone on to take additional training in a more specific area of that specialty. For example, nephrology, which deals with the kidneys, is a subspecialty of internal medicine; child psychiatry is a subspecialty of psychiatry; and hand surgery is a subspecialty of general surgery. These specialties and subspecialties will be discussed in later chapters in greater detail.

A physician who successfully completes an approved residency program and other requirements may elect to take an examination offered by the specialty board that issues certificates in that specialty or subspecialty. Some specialty boards have written and oral exams. Physicians who pass the exam(s) become board certified, if they meet the other criteria of that specialty board. Physicians do not have to be board certified to practice medicine, but some hospitals do require it. Board certification is sometimes necessary for eligibility for certain types of liability insurance, or for membership in some specialty societies.

LOCATION OF RESIDENCY PROGRAMS

Most residency programs are situated in hospitals. Residency programs might also exist in ambulatory clinics, outpatient surgical centers, mental health clinics or agencies, public health agencies, blood banks, medical examiners' offices, or physicians' offices.

Geographically, residency programs tend to be in densely populated areas of the country. The residency program's goal is to expose the new physician to as many medical or surgical situations as possible. Rural settings have less variety than urban ones and don't give the resident, especially in certain specialties and subspecialties, as rich and diverse a clinical experience. New York has the most residency programs, and California ranks second.

MINORITIES AND WOMEN IN RESIDENCIES

In 1988 there were over 81,000 residents on duty in the United States. Of these, 80 percent were Caucasian. Less than 5 percent of the total resident population was black. The majority of black residents were in internal medicine, surgery, obstetrics and gynecology, family practice, and pediatrics.

Another 5 percent of residents were Hispanic, mostly Mexican American and Puerto Rican. The remaining 10 percent were Asian, Pacific Islander, American Indian, or Alaskan native.

Also in 1988, 28 percent of all residents were women. Women are most concentrated in internal medicine, pediatrics, and family medicine.

HOURS WORKED

Everyone has heard stories of the number of hours that residents work. In fact, there has been a great deal of media attention lately about the legendary hours that residents work. The data supports the legend.

The number of hours worked and the stress involved in being a resident have been causes of concern for years. A recent court case concerning a patient's death held that the patient died because the resident involved was inadequately supervised and fatigued by excessive work hours.

The case was well-publicized. It brought the general public into the ongoing concern about problems associated with the heavy work load residents in certain programs must sometimes bear. Some changes are already being made, and others are being looked at in response to those concerns.

The American Medical Association (AMA) conducted a survey to see how many hours residents worked in 1987. On the average, including all specialties, residents spent over 74 hours a week in their residency programs. Over 58 hours a week were spent in patient care. Almost seven hours a week were spent receiving some type of formal instruction, and four hours a week were spent teaching other residents and medical students. Research and administrative duties each took less than three hours a week. Average number of nights spent on-call each month for all residents in 1987 was eight.

The number of hours worked varies dramatically from specialty to specialty. Table 3.1 is taken from the 1987 Survey of Resident Physicians, done by the AMA Center for Health Policy Research. This table shows the average number of hours worked by residents in selected specialties. The table includes the average for all years of residency training, and the average number of hours worked in the first year of training, which is always higher.

Table 3.1

Specialty	*Average Hours Worked Weekly*	
	First Year	*All Years*
Family Practice	82.3	70.5
Internal Medicine	90.3	74.6
Surgery	98.0	87.0

Specialty	Average Hours Worked Weekly	
	First Year	All Years
Pediatrics	93.6	70.2
Obstetrics/Gynecology	93.9	89.1
Radiology	51.0	50.1
Psychiatry	66.5	52.6
Anesthesiology	81.4	76.0
Pathology	54.3	47.9
Other	87.3	71.0

This does not include moonlighting, which is extra work that residents may take to make extra money.

FINANCES

By the time a physician graduates from medical school, he or she often has accumulated a great debt. For students who had debt, in 1988 the average amount owed was $38,489. Twenty-four percent of the students with debt owed over $50,000.

Residents do receive salary and benefits, but sometimes feel they have to moonlight to either make ends meet or to begin to repay their debt.

In 1987, the average annual salary of residents was $24,361. In that same year, over 37 percent of all residents were involved in moonlighting. These residents spent an average of over 13 hours per week moonlighting. Average income earned from these activities was $7,100.

Benefits are also included in residency programs. Most residents get health insurance and liability insurance as part of their benefits package. Many residents also get meals and parking as a part of the benefits they receive. Less often, residents receive housing and child care as part of the benefits package.

THE FUTURE OF GRADUATE MEDICAL EDUCATION

Graduate medical education will undergo many changes in the future. The face of medicine is changing (the final chapter discusses this in greater detail), and these changes will affect the way physicians are trained. The numbers of women entering the medical profession and their concerns will affect residency training as well. For example, shared-schedule residencies, which exist now, but not in great numbers, are likely to become more prominent. Shared-schedule residencies are those in which a single position is shared by two people, but the length of the residency is increased. This enables those sharing the position to pursue other interests or commitments, such as parenting, with a less demanding training schedule.

The aging of America, the concerns about overly rigorous residency schedules, new regulations set by the government, and breakthroughs in understanding health and disease will continue to change the way physicians will learn to treat patients in the future.

CHAPTER 4

FAMILY PRACTICE AND GENERAL INTERNAL MEDICINE

The old time GP, or general practitioner, is a relic of the past, but the medical specialty of family practice has stepped in to take its place. Internal medicine physicians, often called internists, are specialists, too, and also often serve as a person's main, or primary care, physician. That means that these two specialties have some overlap. In this chapter, we'll look at the philosophy, training, practice, and salary of these two specialties to see what they have in common and how they differ.

FAMILY PRACTICE

Background

After World War II, medical specialties began to expand rapidly. While in 1940 three out of four physicians were general practitioners, by 1949 only two out of three were general practitioners.

Medicine was changing. Medical staffs were beginning to require board certification for physicians with hospital privileges. Residency programs in family practice were very limited, too. Even internal medicine was a specialty. So as the specialists gained status and popularity, the general practitioner was left behind.

When the general practitioners began to take action on their diminishing status, they saw that one of the hallmarks of their style of medicine was the interaction with patients and their families. So, the terms family physician and family practice began to emerge. By 1969, family practice was a board certified specialty.

The Profession

The family practitioner provides health care in medicine and surgery from prenatal care to geriatric, or old age, care. The family physician is trained to provide comprehensive and continuing care, also called primary care, often to entire families, regardless of sex, age, or type of problem. If a problem is beyond the scope of a family physician, he or she will refer to another physician who specializes in the particular problem.

Even if a family physician does not treat a whole family, he or she always approaches medicine within the context of a family. In other words, a family practitioner always takes the patient's family into consideration. That means emphasis on the kinds of disease patterns found within a family, and even attention paid to family life-style.

Medical students are often attracted to family practice because of the diversity of the field. They can diagnose and treat, and be around to see a patient's continuing progress.

Close and continuing relationships are also an attractive part of the family practice specialty. Most family physicians would define themselves as "people persons" who enjoy the close contact with their patients.

Because they are specialists who deal with a range of problems, from physical to emotional to social, they can offer care that takes into account the total person. Many patients are seeking this type of care today.

Their wide range of skills also brings family physicians into direct competition for patients with other physicians. The specialties that they most often overlap with are internal medicine, obstetrics and gynecology, and pediatrics.

Every specialty has its drawbacks, and family practice is no exception. Because of the nature of the care they provide, family physicians put in long hours. Because of their close relationships with patients, family practitioners are called a lot and sometimes have interrupted personal lives as a result.

Despite the long hours and hard work, family physicians make less money than other physicians. The average annual gross income for all physicians is approximately $210,000. The average gross income of a family physician is approximately $140,000.

All self-employed physicians must pay liability insurance. The average liability premium a year for all physicians in 1988 was $15,900; the average premium for family physicians was $9,400.

Training

In 1970, there were only 49 approved residency programs in family practice; by 1988, there were 382. The American Board of Family Practice requires successful completion of a three-year residency program. The only prerequisite for entry to a residency program in family practice is the completion of the M.D. degree.

Residents get experience with both inpatients (patients who are staying in the hospital) and outpatients (patients who are not hospitalized). As the three years progress, residents take increasing responsibility for all aspects of patients' care.

In addition, family practice training emphasizes preventive medicine, community medicine, and application of understanding of human behavior to the day-to-day practice of medicine. Family practice was the first specialty board requiring periodic recertification, using a written test at six-year intervals.

In response to the aging population and to the number of family practice-based geriatric programs, the American Board of Family Practice in 1985 added an additional certificate program for physicians with an interest in geriatrics. Fellowship programs based in family practice residencies are also available—in geriatrics, obstetrics, sports medicine, and other clinical and educational areas.

INTERNAL MEDICINE

Background

The words "internal medicine" were used by German physicians late in the nineteenth century to describe a branch of medicine which did not use surgical methods of treatment with patients.

The American Congress on Internal Medicine was established in 1915 to facilitate exchange of ideas among physicians interested in this branch of medicine, to publish, and to grant research fellowships. This group became today's professional association, the American College of Physicians, which had 65,000 members in 1988.

The Profession

Specialists in internal medicine primarily treat adults. Some treat adolescents, as well. Internists, as they are often called, intimately understand all the major organ systems. Internists diagnose and treat acute and chronic diseases, usually from practices based in offices. They also see patients hospitalized for problems that fall under the domain of internal medicine.

Internists have a wide range of patients from those who are very healthy to those with serious illnesses. In a day, an internist may treat colds, flu, and sore throats and also treat diabetes, heart problems, and AIDS.

In medical school, it is often said that internal medicine is an intellectual medical specialty because internists often diagnose and treat based on discussion with their patients rather than relying on extensive batteries of tests and procedures that help them discover the problem.

Some internists are board certified in internal medicine and another internal medicine specialty such as cardiology or gastroenterology. This enables these physicians to have a general internal medicine practice, but also to be experts in a particular aspect of internal medicine.

Like family practice, internal medicine offers close and long-term relationships with patients. An internist is often in charge of overall patient management because of this relationship. If a patient has a problem that requires specialty treatment, the internists often coordinate that care. Internal medicine can be a challenging specialty because of the diversity and intellectual stimulation it offers.

However, like family practitioners, internists must have a high degree of availability. They therefore may sacrifice more of their personal lives than physicians in some other specialties.

Despite the long hours and degree of responsibility, internists are not among the highest paid physicians. Their average annual gross income is approximately $185,000. Their liability premiums tend to be lower than many other physicians, however. In 1988, internists paid an average of $9,000, just a little lower than family practitioners.

Training

Residency training for general internal medicine is three years long. The prerequisite to training is the completion of the M.D. degree. In 1988 there were 442 accredited residency programs in internal medicine. Board certification is granted through the American Board of Internal Medicine.

There has been a decrease over the last five years in the number of internal medicine residency positions filled by U.S. medical school graduates. The factors for this decrease are numerous. They include a decrease in the number of U.S. medical school graduates and an increase in the total number of residency positions in internal medicine.

Also, the newer reimbursement mechanisms for primary care physicians, such as internists, are not as good as they are in some other subspecialties. Reimbursement mechanisms are the rates at which insurance companies and the government reimburse doctors and patients for medical treatment and procedures. Interviewing patients and diagnosis, which are a large part of a primary care practice, are often not reimbursed at as high a rate as procedures that are more technological in nature. Therefore, this reimbursement system may be creating a financial disincentive for students to become primary care physicians, such as internists or family practitioners.

Because of problems in the past with overly long working hours and exceptionally strenuous work load, the Residency Review Committee in Internal Medicine has established new residency program accreditation standards effective in 1989. New standards address such items as hours, which are stipulated as no more than 80 hours per week, and the range of patients for which a first-year resident in internal medicine should be responsible.

Beyond general internal medicine, there are many subspecialties and certificates that a person wishing to specialize further can obtain. These subspecialties will be discussed in the next chapter.

CHAPTER 5

MEDICAL SPECIALISTS

Internal medicine has many branches which probe into either organ systems, a particular age group, or another area of expertise. These branches are called subspecialties. Each of these subspecialties formerly dealt only with nonsurgical procedures, although in some specialties that has changed, and will be noted in the description. As medicine progresses, new subspecialties will be added to the list. In fact, some subspecialties are so new that little or no data is available. In those cases, a brief description of the subspecialty will be given. Average annual salaries are not available for the internal medicine subspecialties. Average annual gross income for all nonsurgical specialists is around $185,000, however.

CARDIOVASCULAR MEDICINE

Cardiovascular diseases are the leading cause of death in the United States. Therefore, the subspecialist in cardiovascular medicine—the cardiologist—has a wide ranging and important job to do.

Cardiology is the subspecialty dedicated to diagnosing and treating diseases and malfunctions of the heart, lungs, and blood vessels. It is a highly challenging and intellectual discipline of medicine, combining diagnostic mastery with a knowledge of highly technological procedures.

Because they are heart specialists, cardiologists treat a significant population of elderly people. And because of the significance of the heart in the human body, cardiologists deal, more than some other specialists, in chronic illness and life-and-death emergencies.

Although in past years cardiology was primarily a diagnostic and medically oriented specialty, in more recent years advances in the field have demanded more invasive procedures. An example of this trend is cardiac catheterization, where a patient, under local anesthetic in an operating room, has dye injected into the arteries so that the cardiologist may locate any blockages. This type of complicated, invasive procedure has brought some cardiologists closer to being surgeons than they were before. As a result, cardiologists now divide themselves into two groups, invasive and noninvasive, depending upon how they practice the subspecialty. Common conditions that cardiologists treat include coronary artery disease, heart attacks, hypertension, life-threatening abnormal heart rhythms, and stroke.

In addition to diagnosis and high-tech intervention, cardiologists also place a high premium on prevention and are on the forefront of the preventive medicine frontier. Advances in knowledge about nutrition and exercise have helped reduce the number of deaths from heart disease.

Medical students who are interested in cardiology are often attracted by the challenge of this quickly evolving field. It is a subspecialty where diagnosis, high-tech progress, and prevention all meet. Cardiologists have a combination of long-term relationships with some patients and consultative roles with others.

Cardiology can be a stressful area of medicine because of the nature of its subject. Sometimes cardiologists deal with very sick people who cannot be helped. And because of the life-and-death aspects of their subspecialty, cardiologists often deal with problems that can't wait, which can interrupt the cardiologist's personal life.

There were 226 accredited programs in cardiology in 1988. Training in cardiology includes three years of a general internal medicine residency with two additional years of training in cardiology. In 1993, the two-year requirement in cardiology will expand to three years, with the general internal medicine requirement remaining.

Although there has been steady growth in the number of cardiologists, the increasing elderly population is likely to increase the demand for cardiologic services in the future.

Most cardiologists have practices from which they treat patients.

In the past most cardiologists' practices were solo practices. There has been a shift recently toward group practices. About one-third of a cardiologist's time with patients is spent in hospital rounds. Many of their hospitalized patients are in special units called coronary care, or cardiac units. A small percentage are researchers only, and there are many opportunities for cardiologists in research.

ENDOCRINOLOGY AND METABOLISM

Endocrinologists manage the diagnosis and treatment of the hormone-producing glandular and metabolic systems. Endocrinologists treat a diverse age range, see a wide variety of diseases, and have patients who range from very sick to those who need brief treatment. In addition to seeing patients, endocrinologists often do research, blending the two disciplines of clinical medicine and research more than many other specialties.

Endocrinology requires broad knowledge of other fields of medicine and often has positive outcomes. Endocrinologists treat such disorders as thyroid conditions, diabetes, pituitary disorders, calcium disorders, sexual problems, nutritional disorders, and hypertension. Because of the nature of some of the diseases they treat, such as diabetes, there is a lot of opportunity for endocrinologists to use an educational component in their treatment, teaching patients with an ongoing condition how to manage their illnesses.

Endocrinologists work long hours. However, the analytical nature of the subspecialty is what attracts medical students and residents. And, although endocrinologists don't always know the outcomes of their patients' illnesses, their emphasis on analytic reasoning is a positive force in the field. Rapidly developing technology in endocrinology also challenges those pursuing it.

In 1988 there were 140 accredited training programs in endocrinology. Three years of internal medicine are required with an additional two years in endocrinology and metabolism.

GASTROENTEROLOGY

Gastroenterology deals with the diagnosis and treatment of disorders of, or relating to, the digestive system. This includes the stomach, bowels, liver, gallbladder, and related organs. Gastroenterologists treat such diseases as cirrhosis of the liver, hepatitis, ulcers, cancer, jaundice, inflammatory bowel disease, and irritable bowel disease. Their caseloads are mostly made up of adults and the elderly. Infants and children form a very small percentage of their patient populations.

Gastroenterology is a procedures-oriented specialty and, as such, a high degree of motor skill and manual dexterity is required. But there is medical investigation as well, and gastroenterologists enjoy a good mix of patient care, diagnostic challenges, and procedures.

Some gastroenterologists say that a frustrating part of their field is dealing with patients who do not comply with treatments and patients who wait so long for treatment that nothing can be done. Some also mind that some of the procedures they must do are physically uncomfortable for their patients. These procedures include endoscopy, where the physician visualizes the hollow organs through lighted endoscopes. Through these endoscopes, the gastroenterologist can biopsy tissues and remove small growths.

Because of invasive procedures like endoscopy, the field of gastroenterology is more surgical than it used to be. Gastroenterologists' level of responsibility is very high because of the invasiveness of some of the procedures they perform.

Gastroenterology is a lucrative field, although the hours are long, and there are emergency consultations on nights and weekends.

In 1988 there were 184 accredited training programs in gastroenterology. Gastroenterologists must finish three years of training in internal medicine and complete another two years in gastroenterology.

HEMATOLOGY

Hematology is the subspecialty which deals with blood and blood diseases. Hematologists also deal with the spleen and lymph glands. Hematologists are researchers in addition to clinicians. Many hematology training programs are connected to medical oncology programs. Oncology relates to cancer.

Hematologists treat all organ systems, but always related to the blood in those systems. They treat all age groups. Medical advances in this field continue to grow rapidly, and diagnosis and treatment often involve use of high-tech equipment.

Blood diseases are often serious or fatal, and physicians pursuing this field must be prepared for the stresses of dealing with critically ill patients. Hematologists can, however, improve the quality of their patients' lives. Hematologists treat leukemia, other cancers of the blood, lymphoma, sickle cell disease, hemophilia, serious anemia, and secondary problems that arise when a patient has another type of cancer. They also perform blood transfusions and biopsies on bone marrow.

Like many other subspecialties of internal medicine, hematology is very analytical and intellectually demanding, and physicians considering this subspecialty must be attracted and challenged by those rigors. And, because of the research and writing involved in hematology, it is a valuable asset if the person choosing this field is a good writer.

Hematologists must deal with the ongoing strains of death, even in the young, but not lose their compassion in the process. Because of the demanding nature of this subspecialty, personal time can be limited.

There were 157 accredited training programs in hematology in 1988. Hematologists must finish three years of training in general internal medicine and complete another two years in a hematology training program. The U.S. Department of Health and Human Services reports that there will be a deficit of hematologists in the 1990s.

INFECTIOUS DISEASES

Subspecialists in infectious disease diagnose and treat communicable disease. In the past, most of those practicing this subspecialty worked at hospitals or medical centers where difficult cases would be referred. Today, however, there are more opportunities for private practice in this field. Infectious disease specialists are usually found in cities because they need to have referrals from a large number of other physicians in order to thrive in their work.

The pursuit of infectious diseases is again intellectually challenging and requires some detective work for excellence. People are usually referred to these specialists when other physicians can't determine the cause of the problem, or the problem is either so specialized or so rare that it warrants referral. For instance, when a person has a fever and it cannot be explained by anyone, the patient is often referred to an infectious disease specialist. This makes the field of infectious diseases especially diverse.

One facet of this specialty has changed dramatically in recent years: the advent of AIDS. This aspect of the infectious disease specialist's practice can be very stressful because, as of now, AIDS is always fatal and often strikes young people.

As in many other internal medicine subspecialties, infectious diseases is not procedures oriented. Therefore, infectious disease specialists are not compensated as well as the more procedures oriented specialists. Diseases that these specialists treat range from rare, tropical diseases to AIDS to pneumonia. As infectious diseases are transmitted from person to person, usually through some form of contact, there is also a public health aspect to this subspecialty when outbreaks occur and affect whole populations of people. Most infectious disease specialists do not form long-lasting relationships with patients who are referred to them for one problem. The notable exception is in the case of AIDS, where the infectious disease specialist sometimes becomes the primary care physician.

There were 150 accredited training programs in infectious diseases in 1988. Three years of internal medicine residency are mandatory followed by at least two years of subspecialty training in infectious diseases.

MEDICAL ONCOLOGY

Medical oncology deals with tumors and cancers which occur in all organ systems. This subspecialty is closely related to hematology. It is a multidisciplinary field because the medical oncologist treats all organ systems. Therefore, oncologists often consult with specialists in those systems. Because there has been such an explosion of knowledge about cancer, oncology is a rapidly expanding, and ever-changing discipline. Research opportunities in oncology are plentiful.

Because of the nature of this field, oncologists who primarily treat patients must face the problems associated with close contact with seriously or terminally ill patients. There is a high patient mortality rate, and each person entering this field must work out ways of remaining a good physician while dealing with death much more than most other physicians. It is important in oncology to have a support system of one's own to help ease the emotional stress.

The nature of this subspecialty, however, provides lots of opportunities for getting to know patients well and having a high degree of involvement in their lives. Medical oncologists are often very involved with patients' families, too.

Because no two cases are alike, and because all organ systems are involved, the field of oncology is very diverse. Oncologists work on specific, practical problems and also examine larger, more theoretical issues. They are required to know a great deal about all aspects of medicine. Oncologists depend upon referrals from other physicians. They spend most of their hours during the week in patient care.

There were 159 training programs in oncology in 1988. After a three-year residency in general internal medicine, an additional two years of subspecialty training in oncology are required.

NEPHROLOGY

Nephrology deals with diseases and malfunctions of the kidneys and the urinary system. Nephrologists treat kidney disorders, fluid and mineral imbalances, renal failure, and diabetes. They are involved with dialysis and consultation with surgeons about kidney transplantation.

Nephrologists see chronically ill patients and have an extremely focused specialty with an excellent and broad-based knowledge of general internal medicine. Nephrologists can help chronically ill patients lead more productive lives. However, like some other subspecialists in general internal medicine, they must also face the challenges of treating some very sick patients. Many nephrologists have patients who wait patiently for many years for a kidney to become available for transplantation.

Nephrologists, because they treat chronic diseases, get to know patients well and have lots of contact with patients' families. There is a high level of continuous care in this field.

Like many other subspecialties of internal medicine, nephrology is as diverse as it is intellectually challenging. Many facets of science and medicine are applied in nephrology: the basic sciences, chemistry, physics, and good people skills.

There were 152 accredited training programs in nephrology in 1988. Along with a three-year residency in general internal medicine, an additional two-year residency is required in nephrology.

PULMONARY MEDICINE

Pulmonary medicine deals with the treatment of disorders of the respiratory system. Pulmonary specialists, called pulmonologists, treat the lungs and other chest tissues. Pulmonologists treat cancer, pneumonia, occupational diseases, bronchitis, emphysema, asthma, and other lung disorders. They may test lung functions, probe into the bronchial airways, and manage mechanical breathing assistance. Pulmonologists often are found in departments of hospitals called critical care units.

There is a lot of variety in pulmonary medicine, and pulmonologists consult with patients, do many procedures, and practice high-tech interventions. They see patients in practices but also spend a great deal of time in the hospital. As in many of the subspecialties in internal medicine, the hours are very long. Because of the nature of their specialty, pulmonologists spend a lot of time in consultation with other physicians.

In 1988 there were 177 accredited programs in pulmonary medicine. After a three-year residency in general internal medicine, an additional two years of training in pulmonary medicine are required.

RHEUMATOLOGY

Rheumatologists diagnose and treat joint, muscle, and skeletal problems. Arthritis, muscle strains, athletic injuries, and back pain are some of the diseases that rheumatologists treat. They also deal with autoimmune diseases, such as lupus, which may have rheumatologic symptoms.

This is a rapidly evolving field. Rheumatologists are involved in prevention because some of the diseases they treat have been linked, at times, to life-style or nutritional problems. Because of the chronic nature of many of the diseases they treat, rheumatologists tend to have long-term, close relationships with their patients. Many rheumatologists say it is important to have good listening ability and compassion as many of the diseases they treat, such as rheumatoid arthritis, are very painful. Rheumatologists are, to a higher degree than some other subspecialties in internal medicine, extremely involved in the management of pain.

Rheumatologists can have more regular hours than many of their colleagues because there is little critical care involved. Many rheumatologists have office-based practices.

In 1988 there were 116 accredited programs in rheumatology. Three years of residency in general internal medicine are required along with an additional two years of training in rheumatology.

OTHER SUBSPECIALTIES

Other areas of internal medicine include newer subspecialties. Less data is available about the newer subspecialties than exists for more established fields. Three of these new subspecialties are critical care medicine, geriatric medicine, and diagnostic laboratory immunology.

Critical Care Medicine

Critical care medicine involves management of life-threatening, acute disorders—mostly in intensive care units. Critical care specialists take care of patients with shock, coma, heart failure, respiratory arrest, drug overdoses, massive bleeding, diabetic acidosis, and kidney shutdowns. Critical care is a subspecialty of these specialty boards: internal medicine, anesthesiology, neurological surgery, obstetrics and gynecology, and general surgery.

Geriatric Medicine

Although most subspecialties treat the elderly, geriatric medicine offers physicians the opportunity to intimately understand the needs of the elderly. Greater longevity has increased the incidence of chronic and disabling conditions among the elderly. Many older people are on more than one drug, and the drug interaction must be recognized. Diseases are different when they affect older people, and the geriatric specialist is familiar with those differences. Geriatric care specialists also understand how to use resources such as nursing homes and social services for the elderly. The subspecialty of geriatric medicine is sponsored jointly by family practice and internal medicine.

Diagnostic Laboratory Immunology

Diagnostic laboratory immunology is a subspecialty of allergy and immunology, pediatrics, and internal medicine. Diagnostic laboratory immunologists perform laboratory tests and complex procedures that are used to diagnose and treat diseases and conditions resulting from defective immune systems.

CHAPTER 6

SURGERY AND SURGICAL SPECIALTIES

The word "surgeon" was originally "chirurgeon." It came from the Greek word *cheir,* meaning hand, and *ergon,* meaning work. In the seventeenth century, surgeons were socially inferior to other physicians. Very few surgeons had university degrees. While physicians were addressed as "doctor," surgeons were addressed as "mister." Barber surgeons used their razors to open veins for bloodletting, and to trim beards and cut hair.

Surgery has come a long way from the early days in America. Some of these changes are discussed in the first chapter. Today, general surgeons and those in eight other surgical specialties are highly trained, well-respected, and well-paid members of the medical community. In this chapter, we will discuss these nine specialties.

GENERAL SURGERY

General surgery is the specialty that involves all types of surgical operations. Although general surgeons have heavy competition from the other surgical specialties, general surgery remains one of the most popular areas of specialization. In medical school, it is often said that those who go into surgery want clear-cut answers and results. They don't like the ambiguities and gray areas that arise in internal medicine.

A surgeon's hours can be long, irregular, and grueling. Not all surgery is planned or elective, and when a patient needs surgery, the surgeon must be there. This, of course, can happen at any time of the day or night. Surgery is not a specialty that involves many long-term relationships between doctor and patient. Most patients need an operation, and then they improve, no longer needing the surgeon's services. Conditions that a surgeon typically treats are gallbladder disease, hernia, appendicitis, breast cancer, cancers of the digestive system, and emergencies.

The surgeon treats everything from minor health problems to profoundly serious diseases. This aspect of surgery lends a lot of diversity to the profession. Surgeons operate on patients of all ages, but because of the subspecialty of pediatric surgery, in some areas of the country, they treat mostly adults. There is a considerable amount of pressure in all surgical subspecialties because of the nature of the work and the responsibility that is placed upon surgeons.

Average gross annual income of general surgeons is around $235,000 a year. Average annual gross income for all surgical specialties is around $290,000. Surgeons make excellent incomes, but many do have high expenses. Average liability premiums for surgeons were $26,500, for example. (That can be lower in some surgical specialties, but can also be much higher.) Average annual liability premiums for all physicians were $15,900 in 1988.

In 1988 there were 296 accredited residency programs in general surgery. A five-year residency in general surgery is required by the American Board of Surgery.

COLON AND RECTAL SURGERY

Colon and rectal surgeons deal with diseases of the intestinal tract, anus, and rectum. Until 1961 this specialty was called proctology because of the root *proctos,* the Greek word for anus. The name was changed to reflect the broader scope of the specialty.

Colon and rectal surgeons treat all age groups, but middle-aged and older patients predominate. Although they are surgeons, these specialists provide a mix of medical and surgical procedures. An average day may involve some surgery, but also diagnostic techniques such as endoscopy, discussed in chapter 5 under the section on gastroenterology. Colon and rectal surgeons treat hemorrhoids, fissures, polyps, cancer, colitis, and diverticulitis. Many of these diseases and conditions are easy to diagnose, and treatment has a high rate of success.

This ability to diagnose and treat effectively is one of the most positive aspects of becoming a colon and rectal surgeon. There is a lack of emergency situations, which makes colon and rectal surgeons' hours much more within their control than in many other specialties. There is a good diversity of patients, ranging from the uncomfortable to the very sick.

Physicians in this specialty spend time in their offices and time in the hospital. A high degree of manual dexterity is required for this specialty, both because surgery is so exacting and for the diagnostic procedures used. Colon and rectal surgeons can give quick relief to patients who are suffering from painful conditions.

There are opportunities for research in this field. Because they deal with colon and rectal cancer, new techniques for care and preventive measures are constantly being sought. Although their area of expertise is narrowly focused, the prerequisite training in general surgery gives these specialists a good, working knowledge of internal medicine. This is important since many conditions that colon and rectal specialists treat originate elsewhere in the body. The field of gastroenterology is especially related to this field.

Hours in this specialty are fairly regular, making it less demanding than many of the internal medicine subspecialties and some of the other surgical specialties.

There are a small number of training programs, and colon and rectal surgeons have one of the longest training programs in medicine. There were only 27 accredited training programs in 1988. Completion of a five-year program in general surgery is a prerequisite to a one- or two-year residency in colon and rectal surgery. The field is uncrowded with many opportunities for new physicians.

NEUROLOGICAL SURGERY

Neurological surgery, better known as neurosurgery, deals with diagnosis, evaluation, and treatment of disorders of the central, peripheral, and autonomic nervous systems. Practitioners use high-tech equipment such as CT scan and Magnetic Resonance Imaging (MRI) to diagnose problems, along with regular physical examination in the office.

It can be a highly stressful and highly demanding specialty because it deals with the brain. The variation in outcomes is great; there are remarkable interventions and profound disappointments. There can be death or severe disability when the nature of the condition is profound.

The brain is a fascinating organ, and there is much research into the brain. At this point in history, we are just beginning to understand its mysteries. Many neurosurgeons say their work is less a career than a calling, and they do it out of love of the subject.

The threat of malpractice is greater in neurosurgery than in some other specialties, and insurance premiums are extremely high as a result. The hours are long, and because neurosurgeons treat accidents and brain disorders that erupt suddenly, they may be called at any hour of the day. Yet, neurosurgery is challenging, creative, and constantly changing. And, because of the serious nature of the problems neurosurgeons deal with, practitioners get to know their patients well.

Neurosurgeons use their hands extensively, and a good deal of manual dexterity and technical skill is required. Neurosurgeons treat brain and spinal cord cancers, hydrocephalus, lumbar and cervical disc disease, aneurysms, and head and spinal cord trauma. Neurosurgeons must be excellent problem solvers, and they must also understand the logic of anatomy, physiology, and integration of the nervous system.

Neurosurgeons see a wide variety of conditions and serve a range of ages. They move between hospital visits, the operating room, and office settings.

Neurosurgeons rank among the highest paid specialists. The average gross annual income is around $410,000. However, expenses, such as liability premiums, can be very high.

In 1988 there were 93 accredited training programs in neurosurgery. A year of a general surgery residency is required as well as a five-year residency in neurosurgery.

OPHTHALMOLOGY

Ophthalmology is one of several surgical specialties without the word surgeon in its title. Ophthalmology brings surgery, medicine, and diagnostic prowess to the diseases and abnormalities of the eye.

Ophthalmologists deal with sight loss, conjunctivitis, glaucoma, and cataracts. They treat the very young to the very old. Because they work on such a small and delicate part of the body—the eye—ophthalmologists must possess excellent eye-hand coordination and technical skill.

While some of their patients are only seen for one procedure, ophthalmologists have some long-term relationships, with patients who have vision problems, for example. Because they face few life-and-death situations, ophthalmologists deal very little with ethical issues, like the right to die or the rationing of medical care.

Ophthalmologists spend time in office treatment as well as in the operating room. They have some overlap with optometrists, who are not M.D.'s and have their own schools of optometry not related to medical school.

Ophthalmologists' hours are much more controlled than in many other specialties. Annual average gross income is around $360,000.

There were 139 accredited training programs in ophthalmology in 1988. Ophthalmologists must have one year of general residency training, followed by at least three years of an ophthalmology residency.

ORTHOPEDIC SURGEONS

Orthopedic surgery deals with diseased or injured parts of the musculoskeletal system. Practitioners of orthopedic surgery use medicine, surgery, and physical rehabilitation to restore the body to its normal function.

Orthopedic surgeons, sometimes referred to as orthopods, often have broad-based practices, but also may choose a narrower focus such as hand surgery, which is a subspecialty of orthopedic surgery, or sports medicine, which is a subspecialty of family practice. It is often said that orthopedic surgeons are mechanically inclined and like to put things together. The manual dexterity that they need serves not only in microsurgery, delicate spine surgery, and hip replacements, but also serves the practitioner well during casting and manipulation of fractures. Physical strength is also necessary for some procedures.

Conditions that orthopedic surgeons commonly treat include arthritis, fractures, knee trauma, lower back pain, hip trauma, shoulder injuries, deformities, and degenerative diseases of the hip, knees, hand, feet, shoulders, and elbows. Because this specialty often deals with accident victims, there is a certain amount of time spent in assessing disability in legal actions.

One of the most positive aspects about being an orthopedic surgeon is the ability to quickly relieve pain and to see patients leave satisfied and in good condition. There are lots of positive outcomes in orthopedic surgery. Orthopedic surgeons see a wide range of problems and a wide range of patients. It is as common to see children as it is to see the elderly.

Orthopedic surgeons can work very long hours, sometimes 12–15 hours a day. This detracts from a personal life. Their income level, however, is rather high. Annual gross income is around $370,000. But liability premiums are quite high, and the cost of office equipment, such as X-ray machines, is part of the overhead necessary.

In 1989 there were 166 accredited orthopedic training programs. Up to two years are required in a general surgery or other approved medical or surgical residency. Three years are required after that in an orthopedic residency.

OTOLARYNGOLOGY

This specialty of surgery used to be called ENT—ear, nose, and throat, or otorhinolaryngology. In 1980, the name of the specialty was changed to otolaryngology—head and neck surgery. As the title implies, this specialty deals with surgery of the whole head and neck, everything above the shoulders. The exceptions are eye disorders, which are treated by ophthalmologists, and brain disorders, which are treated by neurologists and neurosurgeons.

Otolaryngologists see patients of all ages. Their specialty requires a range of skill because they treat a variety of problems both medically and surgically. Common conditions that otolaryngologists treat include hearing loss, tonsillitis, sinusitis, and head and neck cancers. Their surgical procedures are widely varied because they perform plastic surgery, delicate microsurgery, laser surgery, and major reconstructive procedures.

Otolaryngologists can be in competition with other specialties for patients. The specialties of thoracic surgery, plastic surgery, allergy and immunology, and pulmonary medicine particularly overlap with theirs. Some otolaryngologists solve this by becoming superspecialists, specializing only in facial plastic surgery, for instance, or otology (relating to disorders of the ear).

Otolaryngologists typically have fairly normal working hours and fewer emergencies than many other specialties experience. Annual average gross income is around $320,000.

In 1988 there were 106 accredited training programs in otolaryngology. One or two years of general surgery are required before entering an otolaryngology training program which takes three or four years to complete.

PLASTIC SURGERY

Everyone knows that plastic surgeons make people's noses smaller, reduce wrinkles, and change the shapes of people's bodies. It is a glamorous profession, the province of movie stars and the rich and famous.

What is not as well known is that plastic surgeons also work outside the domain of vanity to restore function to people with deformities, or help burn victims regain a normal appearance. In addition to rhinoplasty for the nose and liposuction for the thighs, plastic surgeons treat a variety of clinical disorders such as cancer, congenital deformities, skin lesions, facial trauma, hand injuries, and degenerative diseases.

It is a highly creative field that requires a good aesthetic sense, attention to detail, and the ability to visualize and imagine. It is also a very innovative field with many new procedures on the horizon like artificial skin for burn patients and fat transfers.

Since plastic surgeons often improve people's appearance or lives, they can gain a great deal of satisfaction from having happy patients. One pitfall in this field can be patients' high or unrealistic expectations. Plastic surgeons see a wide variety of problems and a range of ages. While they sometimes have ongoing relationships with patients, most often they perform one or a few procedures on a patient and the relationship is over.

A high degree of manual dexterity is required. The intellectual demands of the field usually come before the procedure; the plastic surgeon calculates the strategy ahead of time. Plastic surgeons require a combination of resourcefulness, artistic talent, and people skills.

Plastic surgery is very competitive. There are other specialists who perform some of the same procedures, like dermatologists who do skin grafts or otolaryngologists who do face lifts, and this intensifies the competition. There is a great variance in number of hours worked; plastic surgeons who are on-call in a busy emergency room may have long hours, while those who have private practices could have more controllable hours. Average annual gross income for plastic surgeons is around $380,000.

In 1988 there were 97 accredited plastic surgery training programs. The route to becoming a plastic surgeon contains options. Prerequisites are either a three-year residency in general surgery or a residency in otolaryngology or orthopedics. A plastic surgery residency, after the prerequisite is satisfied, lasts at least two years. Many programs require physicians to do three years of plastic surgery if they have not completed residencies in any of the various prerequisite specialties.

THORACIC SURGERY

Thoracic surgery deals with surgery of the chest cavity—the heart, lungs, and esophagus. It is a highly specialized and demanding field and requires decisiveness and the ability to make life-and-death decisions. This specialty demands great manual dexterity and stamina. The hours are long, and the threat of malpractice is greater than in many other specialties.

Common conditions that thoracic surgeons treat are lung cancer, coronary artery disease, aneurysms, and heart disease. While patients of thoracic surgeons can be very ill, surgery can often result in immediate and sometimes dramatic improvement. Thoracic surgeons have a combination of long-term and short-term relationships with patients.

Thoracic surgeons' level of income is high. Average annual gross income is around $325,000. Annual liability premiums are also very high, however.

In 1988, there were 94 accredited training programs in thoracic surgery. It requires the longest residency of any specialty. A five-year general surgery residency is followed by two or three years of a thoracic surgery residency.

UROLOGY

Although urology does not have the word surgeon attached to it, it is, indeed, a surgical specialty. Urology deals with the medical and surgical treatment of disorders of the female urinary tract and the male urogenital tract. Urology relies heavily on diagnostic procedures, and medical intervention can be as significant in treatment as surgery. Common conditions that urologists treat include prostate conditions, malignancies in the genitourinary tract, urinary tract infections, and bladder disorders.

Urologists work with a range of disorders from the very serious to the uncomfortable. Many available interventions can improve dramatically a patient's condition. There are many newer treatments in urology including short, easier treatments for urinary incontinence, prostatic ultrasound, shock wave lithotripsy, and endoscopic surgery. Urologists need coordination and manual dexterity to perform their responsibilities well.

Urologists work primarily with adults and the elderly. They have a high number of long-term relationships with patients. Because they combine medical and surgical treatment, they divide their time between the office and the hospital. Urologists have long hours, but their income is very comfortable. Average annual gross salary is around $250,000.

In 1988 there were 130 accredited training programs in urology. A minimum of five years of residency is required. The first two years are usually in general surgery.

CHAPTER 7

OTHER SPECIALISTS

There are twelve other specialties and many more sub-specialties that were not covered by the preceding chapters. Two of these specialties, pediatrics and obstetrics/gynecology, are primary care specialties. Primary care, as you may recall, is the type of care the patient would seek first. In primary care, patients and their physicians often have ongoing relationships. There are other specialties described in this chapter that many people never have occasion to use.

Anesthesiology, an older specialty, is little understood by the general public. Although everyone knows that these are the doctors who put you to sleep before surgery, very few people understand the intricacies of the profession or the attraction to the profession. Nuclear medicine, on the other hand, is a newer specialty and one that revolves around the exploding technology of the past few decades. The other specialties covered in this chapter are allergy and immunology, dermatology, emergency medicine, pathology, physical medicine and rehabilitation, preventive medicine, psychiatry, and radiology.

PEDIATRICS

Pediatrics is the specialty devoted to the care of infants, children, and teens. Because of the advances in medicine over the past few decades, pediatricians see mostly healthy children and provide well-child care and guidance on prevention of illness.

Pediatrics is a people specialty, and those considering the field should understand that they must like to deal with children and their parents. It is a very demanding branch of medicine and includes long hours and interruptions in the evenings.

Pediatric patients respond well to treatment and are often happy and satisfied customers. Children heal faster than adults, and this aspect of pediatrics can be very gratifying.

In 1985 one in three pediatricians was a woman. The changing life-styles of women will also affect pediatrics in another way: as more women choose to delay or avoid childbearing, the population of children needing services will be reduced.

Although most of their work is with healthy children, pediatricians do see a variety of disorders. These include throat and respiratory infections, communicable diseases, cancer, congenital abnormalities, and developmental and behavioral problems. Pediatricians practice mostly in offices, sometimes in private practice, and sometimes in alternative settings like health maintenance organizations (HMOs). They do make hospital visits, but mainly when they have very ill patients.

Like many of the specialties that are contact-intensive rather than procedures-intensive, pediatricians make less than many of their colleagues. Average annual gross salary is around $170,000. Malpractice premiums are fairly low.

In 1988 there were 234 accredited programs in pediatrics. A three-year residency in pediatrics is required. Subspecialization requires further training. Subspecialties of pediatrics include the following fields.

Pediatric Cardiology. This subspecialty provides comprehensive care from fetal life to young adulthood to patients with cardiovascular disorders.

Pediatric Critical Care. This subspecialist has special competence in advanced life support for children from the newborn to the young adult.

Pediatric Endocrinologist. This subspecialist provides expert care to infants, children, and adolescents who have diseases which stem from the glands that secrete hormones.

Pediatric Hematologist-Oncologist. This subspecialist deals with blood disorders and cancer of the infant, child, teen, and young adult.

Neonatal-Perinatal Medicine. These subspecialists provide care for the sick newborn. They consult with obstetrical colleagues in planning care for infants of high-risk pregnancies, and they consult with pediatricians on the care of the very ill newborn.

*Pediatric Nephrologist.*This subspecialist deals with the normal and abnormal development of the kidney and urinary tract from fetal life to young adulthood.

*Pediatric Pulmonologist.*This subspecialist deals with the prevention and treatment of respiratory diseases affecting infants, children, and young adults.

OBSTETRICS AND GYNECOLOGY

Obstetrics and gynecology (OB/GYN) is a specialty devoted entirely to women. It entails two parts: gynecology, which treats diseases of the female reproductive system, and obstetrics, which deals with the care of women before, during, and after they give birth.

Obstetricians/gynecologists have some interesting issues facing them in today's medical environment. One is that biomedical research has produced profound advances in obstetrical care. These leaps have benefited patients, but have also led to higher, and perhaps unrealistic, expectations among patients. The threat of a malpractice suit is so ever-present that it has led some OB/GYN's to give up the obstetrics part of their practices and just practice gynecology. Others feel that there is too much competition from other professional disciplines, notably family physicians and nurse midwives.

Most OB/GYN patients are healthy. If they are pregnant, their OB/GYN participates in a very important experience and time in their lives. But malpractice premiums, which can amount to over $50,000 a year, are a major issue for this profession today. Lack of sleep, as this is a specialty with erratic hours, and being called out of important personal time, are less appealing facets of this specialty.

Conditions that an OB/GYN might treat other than prenatal care are yeast infections, pelvic pain, endometriosis, infertility, and cancer of the reproductive organs. OB/GYN's are medical doctors and surgeons, and enjoy blending both of those.

Of the 1986 medical school graduates who were planning to enter OB/GYN as a specialty, 69 percent were women, as compared to 34 percent in 1982. This means that the face of OB/GYN will likely shift dramatically in the future from a male-dominated profession to a female-dominated one.

OB/GYN's are many women's primary care specialists and, as such, these specialists have long-term, close, and continuing relationships with their patients. A very small percentage of OB/GYN's include male infertility in their practices, but this is very unusual. This specialty treats women. Good manual dexterity is required because this is a hands-on specialty. OB/GYN's divide their time between the office and the hospital.

OB/GYN's have long, erratic hours and very high expenses, including liability premiums and office and equipment expenses. Average annual gross income is around $290,000.

In 1988 there were 282 accredited training programs in OB/GYN. A four-year residency in obstetrics and gynecology is required. Subspecialization requires two or three years of further training. Subspecialties of OB/GYN include maternal-fetal medicine, which deals with high-risk patients; reproductive endocrinology, which deals with infertility; and gynecologic oncology, which deals with cancers of the reproductive system.

ANESTHESIOLOGY

The American Board of Anesthesiology defines anesthesia as a specialty that deals with the management of patients who are unconscious from causes other than surgery; management of pain relief and problems in cardiac and respiratory resuscitation; application of specific methods of inhalation therapy; and clinical management of various fluid, electrolyte, and metabolic disturbances.

In lay terms, the anesthesiologist manages pain and emotional stress during surgical, obstetrical, and some medical procedures and provides life support under the stress of anesthesia and surgery. Anesthesiologists must have a vast knowledge of physiology and pharmacology.

Many anesthesiologists can choose their own hours. And yet, there is a high level of pressure while they're on the job because they face calls for quick decision making and life-and-death situations. If they are the only anesthesiologist on call at a small but busy hospital, they can have long hours in surgery, and work with a range of health professionals and a range of personalities.

Anesthesiologists spend most of their time in hospitals. This is not a specialty that features close, continuing relationships with patients. Most of an anesthesiologist's contact with patients comes presurgically to evaluate the patient, describe the procedure, and help manage anxiety. Their last encounter with the patient is usually right after surgery.

The surgical procedures that they participate in range from the very routine, like tonsillectomies, to the very complicated, like open heart surgery. This makes their jobs very diverse. There is a reasonable amount of progressive technology in anesthesiology.

The unpredictability of the circumstances makes this a high-pressure field. Average annual gross income is around $215,000, and liability premiums can be fairly high.

In 1988 there were 160 accredited training programs for anesthesiologists. A four-year residency is required for those who specialize in anesthesiology.

NUCLEAR MEDICINE

Nuclear medicine is a young specialty. It is difficult to understand in some ways because it is so highly technological. Nuclear medicine grew out of the fields of radiology, internal medicine, and pathology. It is mainly a diagnostic discipline. For many years X-rays were the only way to see images inside a person's body. Today there is MRI (magnetic resonance imaging) and PET (positron emission tomography), to name a few procedures. These are the domain of nuclear physicians. They are approaches to diagnosis and are opening new vistas in the study of human disease. The word nuclear applied in this way refers to employing the nuclear properties of radioactive and stable nuclides in diagnosis, therapy, and research.

The Joint Commission on the Accreditation of Healthcare Organizations (JCAHO) has stipulated that all hospitals with 300 beds or more should provide nuclear medicine services under the supervision of a qualified nuclear medicine specialist. These procedures are no longer the province only of academic teaching centers. Persons entering this field should be prepared for a rapidly evolving field and should thrive on problem solving.

High-tech equipment is at the core of the nuclear physician's specialty. Therefore, very few nuclear physicians are in private practice because the cost of such equipment is prohibitive. Most practice their specialties within the hospital setting. As a result, they are somewhat constrained by the hospital administration's willingness or ability to keep a department of nuclear medicine up-to-date.

It is often easier to secure a job after residency with the addition of training in radiology. Patient involvement is often limited, so those desiring long-term relationships with patients will not be satisfied with this field. Common conditions that nuclear physicians encounter include thyroid disease, cardiovascular disease, bone pain, and cancer. Most of their patient encounters are with adults and the elderly.

Specialists in this field have flexible hours and a high level of autonomy. Many enjoy the scientific precision with which they can diagnose an illness. Since they diagnose diseases from across the spectrum, there is a high degree of interaction with physicians from other specialties.

There were 91 accredited training programs in nuclear medicine in 1988. A minimum of four years of residency training are necessary to qualify for specialty certification. Two years should be in an approved medical specialty, and two years must be in a nuclear medicine residency.

ALLERGY AND IMMUNOLOGY

Allergy and immunology deals with the human body's reaction to foreign substances. Allergy and immunology was officially designated a specialty in 1972 with the formation of the American Board of Allergy and Immunology. Specialists in this profession follow one of two distinct career paths: clinical practice or academic/research. The field of immunology is experiencing rapid growth, and there are excellent opportunities in the field of immunological research.

Those in clinical practice treat a range of ages from the very young to the very old. They often develop close, long-term relationships with their patients. The majority of their patients are generally healthy. Practitioners in this specialty have regular hours and a distinct lack of emergency cases.

Allergist/immunologists find that certain other specialties also perform some of their procedures. Depending upon which part of the specialty they practice, practitioners from rheumatology, hematology, otolaryngology, or pulmonology may overlap and create competition for allergist/immunologists.

This specialty sees many positive outcomes, and allergist/immunologists can help people suffering from allergic complaints feel much better and get back to leading normal lives. Often entire families have similar patterns of allergies. In this aspect allergist/immunologists are like family practitioners; both sometimes treat the whole family. Since life-style can affect allergies, these practitioners spend some of their time with patients teaching them how to manage their allergies. Conditions that these specialists commonly treat are eczema, asthma, chronic cold symptoms, food and drug allergies, and AIDS.

Even for a physician only involved in clinical practice, this is a diverse field. Because it involves two related but separate disciplines, there is a latitude in the practice. Annual liability premiums are quite low.

In 1988 there were 85 accredited programs in allergy and immunology. Three years of residency in either internal medicine or pediatrics is required before a residency of at least two years in allergy and immunology.

DERMATOLOGY

Dermatology deals with disorders and diseases of the largest organ—the skin. Dermatology deals with minor skin problems such as warts, acne, and eczema. But, it also deals with the removal and biopsy of skin tumors and demands expert diagnostic prowess, for dermatologists are called on regularly by other specialists to help figure out complicated diagnoses. Many dermatologists find they prefer diagnosis, or they prefer a procedure-oriented practice.

Other conditions that a dermatologist commonly treats are psoriasis, all skin cancers, sun damage, and contact dermatitis. Dermatology is a results-oriented profession, and dermatologists do have the benefit of seeing fairly quick results. They typically see fairly healthy patients. The noncritical nature of many dermatological problems facilitates regular working hours.

Dermatologists spend most of their time in office settings. In order to diagnose well, dermatologists must be visually astute. Many diagnoses are made in dermatology on the basis of the way something looks.

Dermatologists have a mix of patient relationships from short-term to long-term. Urban areas tend to be well saturated with dermatologists. Liability premiums are on the low side.

There are a hundred accredited training programs in dermatology. The American Board of Dermatology requires four years of residency training including three years of training in dermatology. Subspecialization requires further training. Dermopathology, and dermatological immunology/diagnostic laboratory immunology are the two subspecialties of dermatology.

EMERGENCY MEDICINE

Emergency medicine is the medical specialty that deals with the immediate decision making and action necessary to prevent further disability or death. Specialists in emergency medicine are found primarily in hospital emergency departments. They are also responsible for setting up emergency medical systems in the hospitals. Because they don't have practices, most emergency room physicians aren't responsible for their own liability insurance; it is often paid for by the hospital. They have very little or no overhead because they don't have offices.

Emergency specialists treat all age groups. They must be prepared to make quick, critical decisions about a patient's welfare, often without a medical history, sometimes when the patient is unconscious. They must be well versed in an infinite variety of illnesses and disorders.

Emergency specialists also must have good interpersonal skills and lots of composure. The hours are usually regular because emergency physicians rotate on a schedule. But most emergency rooms are staffed all night, and this means the emergency physicians often have shifts that are overnight. Switching back and forth from day to night hours can be tough. Holidays and weekends must be staffed in an emergency room as well. Although there is ample time off, shifts can cut into valued personal or family time. Nevertheless, emergency physicians' time off is usually completely free. When they are done with their shifts, they do not have to deal with work until they are there again.

This is not a specialty for those desiring long-term, close relationships with patients. Emergency physicians have no control over who their patients are; they must provide care to anyone who comes through the door. But the decisions and actions that the emergency physician takes can mean the difference between life and death or permanent disability in a person's life.

It is also important to note that some people use emergency rooms as primary care facilities. Therefore, emergency physicians see a good number of nonemergency situations such as flu, strep throat, and twisted ankles. But depending upon the location of their emergency rooms, these physicians also see major trauma like gunshot wounds and bad care accidents.

There were 73 accredited training programs in emergency medicine in 1988. An emergency medicine residency is three years long.

PATHOLOGY

Pathology deals with the causes, manifestations, and diagnoses of diseases. There are two main ways to practice pathology. One is in a hospital, investigating the effects of disease on the human body. These pathologists perform autopsies and examine tissues from patients. This is called anatomical pathology. The other way to practice pathology is as a clinical pathologist. These pathologists work in laboratories supervising testing procedures.

There are several issues of interest facing pathologists today. One is the effect they have felt from the tightening of the belt of government agencies and insurance companies. Most people don't pay for their medical costs entirely alone. But in today's medical environment, it is not as easy to have procedures and services paid for as it was in the past. Continuing efforts to cut costs in health care will affect pathology because most of the diagnostic tests fall into the pathologist's domain. Even a simple blood test is the province of the pathologist once it leaves the doctor's office where it was drawn. It's just that many patients never see the pathologists who help diagnose them.

Also of interest is the exploding technology in pathology. Now, perhaps more than in most periods in history, pathologists can make significant contributions to medicine.

Pathology is not a specialty for those who want relationships with patients. It is a very scientific discipline, and there is little patient contact. There is, however, considerable contact with other specialists. Pathology is diverse, since it spans all medical specialties. Pathologists have regular hours. There can be more business management in pathology than in other specialties. This is because many pathologists have the job of running larger labs.

In 1988 there were 237 accredited programs in pathology. The American Board of Pathology offers certification either in anatomic or clinical pathology, or both. The combined certification takes five years to complete. Subspecialties of pathology include the following fields.

Blood Banking. A physician specializing in blood banking is responsible for the maintenance of an adequate blood supply, blood donor and patient-recipient safety, and appropriate blood utilization. The blood-banking specialist directs the preparation and safe use of specially prepared blood components, including red blood cells, white blood cells, platelets, and plasma constituents.

Chemical Pathology. These specialists deal with the biochemistry of the body as it applies to the cause and progress of disease. This specialty includes the application of biochemical data to the detection, confirmation, or monitoring of a disease. The chemical pathologist often serves as a consultant in the diagnosis and treatment of disease.

Dermopathology. This specialty diagnoses and monitors diseases of the skin. The dermopathologist often serves as a clinical consultant and must have an in-depth knowledge of dermatology, microbiology, parasitology, new technology, and laboratory management.

Forensic Pathology. A forensic pathologist deals with the investigation and evaluation of cases of sudden, unexpected, suspicious, and violent death as well as other specific classes of death defined by law. Quincy, of the old television series, was a forensic pathologist. This specialist sometimes serves the public by becoming a coroner or medical examiner.

*Hematology/Pathology.*This subspecialist deals with diseases that affect the bone marrow, blood cells, blood clotting mechanisms, and lymph nodes. He or she functions as a consultant to all physicians.

*Immunopathology.*This subspecialist is concerned with the scientific study of the causes, the diagnosis, and prognosis of disease using the application of immunological principles to the analysis of tissues, cells, and body fluids.

*Medical Microbiology.*This subspecialist devotes expertise to the isolation and identification of microbial agents that cause infectious diseases. This subspecialist frequently serves as a consultant to primary care physicians when they are dealing with patients with infectious diseases.

*Neuropathology.*Neuropathologists deal with the diagnoses of diseases of the nervous system and muscles; they often serve as consultants to neurologists and neurosurgeons.

PHYSICAL MEDICINE AND REHABILITATION

Physical medicine and rehabilitation (PM & R), also called physiatry, deals with diagnosing, evaluating, and treating patients with impairments and disabilities that involve musculoskeletal, neurologic, cardiovascular, and other body systems. The focus is on the restoration of physical, psychological, social, and vocational function and on alleviation of pain.

Physiatry is a broad field and a new one. There are many opportunities right now in this profession, both in practice and in research. Some physiatrists work in inpatient hospital settings helping to restore stroke or accident victims to a functioning life. This type of practice demands knowledge of, and intersects with, many interesting areas of medicine including orthopedics, neurology, psychiatry, internal medicine, urology, and geriatrics. Other physiatrists have private practices and specialize further in areas like sports medicine.

A high degree of patient and family contact are typical in physiatry. The hours are regular. There is considerable opportunity for patient education, and there can be a great deal of satisfaction inherent in watching the progress that patients make. In addition to those conditions that already have been mentioned, physiatrists also treat arthritis, amputations, back and neck pain, and head and spinal cord trauma.

In 1988 there were 71 accredited training programs in physical medicine and rehabilitation. One year of a general internal medicine residency is required before a physical medicine and rehabilitation residency of three years can be entered.

PREVENTIVE MEDICINE

Preventive medicine is a broad field encompassing general preventive medicine, public health, occupational medicine, and aerospace medicine. It requires knowledge and skill in management, epidemiology, health education and health policy, nutrition, biostatistics, and health services administration. Physicians in this field work in the armed forces, general and family practice, government, hospitals, and industry.

This is not a specialty that includes a lot of people contact. Using the preventive frame of reference, the community is the patient, and the physician's focus is on treating the causes of disease. These causes can include environmental factors, life-style, nutrition, or behavior. These specialists are in the public eye because they help make health policy decisions.

An interesting part of this specialty is that it often deals with people outside the health arena, such as politicians, lawyers, and economists. There is a community-wide or even global approach to this type of medicine, so the gains that are made have the potential to help thousands or even millions of people. Issues that preventive medicine specialists deal with include sexually transmitted diseases, obesity, cholesterol problems, teen pregnancy, environmental hazards, and smoking.

In 1988 the number of accredited training programs was 30 for general preventive health, 25 for occupational health, 9 for public health, and 3 for aerospace medicine. One year of clinical training is a prerequisite to entering residency in preventive medicine. Residency typically includes one academic year leading to a master's degree in public health, or equivalent degree, and one to two years of training in the field. Advanced training may focus on public health, general preventive medicine, occupational medicine, or aerospace medicine. Completion of a residency plus a fourth year of training is required in each of the subspecialties by the American Board of Preventive Medicine.

PSYCHIATRY

Psychiatrists diagnose and treat mental, emotional, and behavioral disorders. Although they have the same medical school training as other physicians, they often use some form of discussion as the basis for treatment. This can take the form of individual therapy or group therapy. Lately, however, there have been great advances in the understanding of the biochemical effects of behavior. As a result, pharmacologic interventions are being used more and more often to treat emotional problems.

Psychiatry is most definitely a people profession. Psychiatrists, more than any other practitioners of medicine, must use all their knowledge to understand the patient's point of reference. Psychiatry is much different than other forms of medicine because at its core it centers on a patient's beliefs, values, and goals.

Psychiatry is an intellectually challenging and reflective profession. It demands that the practitioner challenge his or her own beliefs regularly. There can be a great deal of satisfaction in seeing patients gain confidence and improve their lives.

However, some patient's conditions are chronic, and the person considering psychiatry must learn to live with the fact that some patients will never get fully well. Some conditions like Alzheimer's and schizophrenia create long-term problems. Other conditions that psychiatrists treat include depression, anxiety, personality disorders, and chemical and alcohol dependency.

Psychiatrists who are self-employed can set their own hours. Therefore, their hours are controllable. Gross annual average income is around $140,000. Liability premiums are quite low.

In 1988 there were 206 accredited training programs in psychiatry. The American Board of Psychiatry and Neurology requires a broad-based first year of clinical training followed by a three-year residency in psychiatry. Additional training is required for the subspecialties, such as child psychiatry and geriatric psychiatry.

RADIOLOGY

Radiology deals with diagnosis and treatment of disease using radium-based substances and instruments. Radiologists formerly were trained in both diagnosis and treatment, but today separate programs exist for each of these aspects of practice.

Radiologists are primarily consultants. The diagnostic radiologists use X-rays and other forms of radiant energy to assist other physicians in diagnosing disease. Both types of radiology are mostly hospital based. Rapidly expanding technology demands that radiologists constantly update their knowledge to embrace an ever-expanding constellation of diagnostic and treatment techniques.

Although radiologists do have contact with patients, there is little long-term care involved in radiology. Conditions that radiologists commonly deal with are gastrointestinal complaints, cardiovascular disease, cancers, pulmonary disease, trauma, and hypertension. The hours are fairly regular, as radiologists are mostly behind the scenes in medicine. Average annual gross income is around $220,000.

In 1988 there were 213 accredited programs in diagnostic radiology, 44 in nuclear radiology, and 85 in therapeutic radiology. A three-year residency in diagnostic radiology is required by the American Board of Radiology. Special competence in diagnostic nuclear and therapeutic radiology also is awarded with additional training and other requirements. The major subspecialties are nuclear radiology and pediatric radiology.

CHAPTER 8

MEDICINE IN THE FUTURE

In 1980, a report was published called the "Report of the Graduate Medical Education National Advisory Committee to the Secretary of Health and Human Services." Popularly known as GMENAC, this report predicted which specialties and subspecialties would be over- and undersupplied in medicine. GMENAC had many detractors. Since that time, it seems that no one is willing to go out on that kind of limb and try to predict the future supply and demand for physicians.

The best predictions about the future of a career as a physician come from what has already begun to happen in medicine. Money flowed freely in the 1970s, and doctors were able to give diagnostic tests and treatment at their own discretion. The 1980s brought an era of tightened fists, an era when Americans were becoming aware of scarce resources and were sensitive to the overuse of energy and shortages of food. Excesses in health care were a target as well. In 1983, Medicare's prospective payment system was enacted. This permanently changed the way hospitals were run. The prospective payment system established DRG's (diagnosis-related groups) as the standard method of reimbursement for federally sponsored patients like senior citizens. With the new system, the federal government reimburses hospitals based on cost averaging, rather than what it really costs to treat a patient. Hospitals often receive far less money than it really takes to treat a patient. In the five years following 1983, there were more than 400 hospital closings nationwide. The poorest areas were hit the hardest. If hospitals weren't getting reimbursed what it cost them to treat patients, many could not survive.

AMBULATORY AND MANAGED CARE CENTERS

Changes in health care delivery systems have begun to change the face of medicine as well. The emergence of new types of ambulatory care centers has taken some business away from hospitals. These clinics, with such names as Emergi-Care, offer some of the same care as emergency rooms, but can also substitute for primary care physicians.

Managed care centers, such as health maintenance organizations (HMO's), continue to proliferate. This type of health care delivery cuts down on the level of familiarity and the interaction between provider and patient. Patients may not always see the same doctor, the number of tests that can be run are limited by the rules, and the amount of time that a patient sees a doctor may also be limited by the rules of the organization.

Most HMO's and other systems like them offer savings to patients, and cost containment has proven to be an important issue in the nineties when the seventies and eighties brought such tremendous increases in health care costs.

OTHER TRENDS

There are new demands for accountability of physicians. The public became restless in the late seventies when there was some feeling that doctors thought they had all the answers. More demands are now made on physicians for recordkeeping and justification of their decisions. Many physicians complain that this has turned their love of medicine and belief in the sanctity of the patient-physician relationship into a endless torrent of paperwork and nonmedical busywork.

But health and well-being are precious commodities, and those who care for our health will always be valued. It just may be that the face of medicine is changing. Once a person-to-person job, the advancing scientific body of knowledge will undoubtedly continue to help develop more and more precise instrumentation for sensitive diagnosis and treatment.

This does not mean that doctors will be replaced; they will not. But they will continue to have adjuncts to their art and science not available before. Some doctors will face greater competition than ever before, not as a result of technology, but from their colleagues and other non-M.D. health professionals.

Many physicians are located in urban areas, and in these areas, some specialties will be oversupplied. This may encourage young physicians to practice in areas that have historically shown shortages, such as rural areas. Also, physicians in urban areas may have fewer patient visits than before because of the intense competition for patients. The explosion in the elderly population that is expected between now and the year 2025 and the persistence of chronic diseases such as AIDS will create a demand for the specialties that serve those populations.

In earlier times, it was common for physicians to graduate from medical school, do a residency, then go into private practice. In the future, it will be more and more common for physicians to join a group or a managed care practice, such as those mentioned earlier in this chapter. Very few graduates can afford to start their own practices with the high costs of start-up, the burden of educational debt, and the high cost of liability premiums.

Our approach to medicine is changing as well. The goal of medicine is to cure disease and relieve suffering. More and more, we look beyond the medical model for answers. Where we used to look for a cure for lung cancer, now we also encourage people to change their life-styles and stop smoking. The high rate of infant mortality cannot only be addressed by physicians because physicians alone cannot provide the answers. Teen pregnancy, inadequate housing, and lack of jobs and education all contribute to the problem. People from other walks of life will have to contribute to the solution as well.

Once we thought of medicine as a panacea. Now we know at its best it is an important and honorable profession. But it does not stand alone. Health and wellness are complicated issues. They have to do with life-style, economic status, geography, age, and a host of other factors. The thinking of different disciplines joined together will provide answers. Doctors are essential to that process.

MAJOR PROFESSIONAL ORGANIZATIONS

This is a listing of the major professional organizations and societies. Some groups have more than one related association, so look through the whole list. If you can't find the organization you need, contact the American Medical Association for assistance.

Aerospace Medical Association
    P.O. Box 26128
    Alexandria, VA 22313-6128
    703-739-2240

American Academy of Allergy and Immunology
    611 East Wells Street
    Milwaukee, WI 53202
    414-272-6071

American Academy of Dermatology
    1567 Maple Avenue
    Evanston, IL 60201
    708-869-3954

American Academy of Family Practitioners
    8880 Ward Parkway
    Kansas City, MO 64114-2797
    816-333-9700

American Academy of Neurology
    2221 University Avenue, SE, Suite 335
    Minneapolis, MN 55414
    612-623-8115

American Academy of Ophthalmology
    655 Beach Street
    P.O. Box 7424
    San Francisco, CA 94120
    415-921-4700

American Academy of Orthopedic Surgeons
    22 South Prospect Avenue
    Park Ridge, IL 60068
    708-823-7186

American Academy of Otolaryngology
    Head and Neck Surgery, Inc.
    1101 Vermont Avenue, NW, Suite 302
    Washington, DC 20005
    202-289-4607

American Academy of Pediatrics
    141 Northwest Point Boulevard
    Elk Grove Village, IL 60009
    708-228-5005

American Academy of Physical Medicine and Rehabilitation
    122 South Michigan Avenue, Suite 1300
    Chicago, IL 60603
    312-922-9366

American Academy of Radiology
    1891 Preston White Drive
    Reston, VA 22091
    701-648-8900

American Association of Neurological Surgeons
    22 South Washington Street, Suite 100
    Park Ridge, IL 60068
    708-692-9500

American College of Cardiology
    9111 Old Georgetown Road
    Bethesda, MD 20014
    301-897-5400

American College of Chest Physicians
    911 Busse Highway
    Park Ridge, IL 60068
    708-698-2200

American College of Colon and Rectal Surgery
    615 Griswold, Suite 1717
    Detroit, MI 48226
    313-961-7880

American College of Emergency Physicians
    P.O. Box 619911
    Dallas, TX 75261
    214-550-0911

American College of Gastroenterologists
    13 Elm Street
    Manchester, MA 01944
    617-927-8330

American College of Nuclear Medicine
    P.O. Box 5887
    Columbus, GA 31906
    404-322-8049

American College of Obstetricians and Gynecologists
    600 Maryland Avenue, SW
    Washington, DC 20024
    202-638-5577

American College of Physicians
    4200 Pine Street
    Philadelphia, PA 19104
    215-243-1200

American College of Preventive Medicine
1015 15th Street, NW, Suite 403
Washington, DC 20005
202-789-0003

American College of Surgeons
55 East Erie Street
Chicago, IL 60611
312-664-4050

American Geriatrics Society
770 Lexington Avenue, Suite 400
New York, NY 10021
212-308-1414

American Heart Association
7320 Greenville Avenue
Dallas, TX 75231
214-373-6300

American Medical Association
515 North State Street
Chicago, IL 60610
312-645-5000

American Medical Women's Association
801 North Fairfax Street
Alexandria, VA 22314
212-533-5104

American Psychiatric Association
14 K Street, NW
Washington, DC 20005
202-682-6000

American Rheumatism Association
17 Executive Park Drive, NE, Suite 480
Atlanta, GA 30329
404-633-3777

American Society for Hematology
6900 Grove Road
Thorofare, NJ 08086
619-845-0003

American Society of Anesthesiologists
515 Busse Highway
Park Ridge, IL 60068
708-825-5586

American Society of Clinical Oncology
435 North Michigan Avenue, Suite 1717
Chicago, IL 60611
312-644-0828

American Society of Internal Medicine
1101 Vermont Avenue, NW, Suite 500
Washington, DC 20005
202-289-1700

American Society of Nephrology
60 Grove Road
Thorofare, NJ 08086
609-848-1000

American Society of Plastic and Reconstructive Surgeons, Inc.
233 North Michigan Avenue, Suite 1900
Chicago, IL 60601
312-856-1818

American Thoracic Society
1740 Broadway
New York, NY 10019
212-315-8700

American Urological Association
1120 North Charles Street
Baltimore, MD 21201
301-727-1100

California Hispanic-American Medical Association
P.O. Box 1089
Arcadia, CA 91066
213-469-8362

College of American Pathologists
7400 North Skokie Boulevard
Skokie, IL 60077
708-677-3500

Endocrine Society
9650 Rockville Pike
Bethesda, MD 20014
301-571-1802

Infectious Diseases Society of America
Office of the Secretary
Yale University School of Medicine
201 LCI
333 Cedar Street
New Haven, CT 06510
203-785-4141

National Medical Association (Association of Black Physicians)
1012 Tenth Street, NW
Washington, DC 20001
202-347-1895

Renal Physicians Association
1101 Vermont Avenue, NW, Suite 500
Washington, DC 20005
202-898-1562

Society of Critical Care Medicine
251 East Imperial Highway
Fullerton, CA 92635
714-870-5243

Society of Nuclear Medicine
136 Madison Avenue
New York, NY 10016
212-889-0717

UNITED STATES MEDICAL SCHOOLS

University of Alabama
  School of Medicine
  Office of Medical Student Services/Admissions
  Box 100-UAB Station
  Birmingham, AL 35294
  205-934-2330

University of South Alabama
  College of Medicine
  Office of Admissions
  Room 2015, Medical Sciences Building
  Mobile, AL 36688
  205-460-7176

University of Arizona
  College of Medicine
  Admissions Office
  Tucson, AZ 85724
  602-626-6214

University of Arkansas
  College of Medicine
  Office of Student Admissions, Slot 551
  4301 West Markham Street
  Little Rock, AR 72205
  501-686-5354

University of California, Davis
  School of Medicine
  Chair, Admissions Committee
  Admissions Office
  Davis, CA 95616
  916-752-2717

University of California, Irvine
  College of Medicine
  Office of Admissions
  E112-Medical Sciences Building
  UCI-College of Medicine
  Irvine, CA 92717
  714-856-5388

University of California, Los Angeles
  UCLA School of Medicine
  Office of Student Affairs
  Division of Admissions
  Center for Health Sciences
  Los Angeles, CA 90024
  213-825-6081

University of California, San Diego
  School of Medicine
  Office of Admissions, M-021
  Medical Teaching Facility
  La Jolla, CA 92093-0621
  619-534-3880

University of California, San Francisco
  School of Medicine, Admissions
  C-200, Box 0408
  San Francisco, CA 94143
  415-476-4044

Loma Linda University
  School of Medicine
  Associate Dean for Admissions
  Loma Linda, CA 92350
  714-824-4467

University of Southern California
School of Medicine
Office of Admissions
1975 Zonal Avenue
Los Angeles, CA 90033
213-342-2552

Stanford University
School of Medicine
Office of Admissions
851 Welch Road, Room 154
Palo Alto, CA 94304-1677
415-723-6861

University of Colorado
School of Medicine
Office of Admissions and Records
Box A054
4200 East Ninth Avenue
Denver, CO 80262
303-270-7676

University of Connecticut
School of Medicine
Office of Admissions and Student Affairs
University of Connecticut Health Center
263 Farmington Avenue
Farmington, CT 06032
203-679-2152

Yale University
School of Medicine
Office of Admissions
367 Cedar Street
New Haven, CT 06510
203-785-2643

George Washington University
    School of Medicine and Health Science
    Office of Admissions
    2300 Eye Street, NW
    Washington, DC 20037
    202-994-3506

Georgetown University
    School of Medicine
    Office of Admissions
    3900 Reservoir Road, NW
    Washington, DC 20007
    202-687-1154

Howard University
    College of Medicine
    Admissions Officer
    520 W Street, NW
    Washington, DC 20059
    202-636-6270

University of Florida
    College of Medicine
    Chairman, Medical Selection Committee
    Box J-216
    J. Hillis Miller Health Center
    Gainesville, FL 32610
    904-392-3071

University of Miami
    School of Medicine
    Office of Admissions
    P.O. Box 016159
    Miami, FL 33101
    305-547-6791

University of South Florida
  College of Medicine
  Office of Admissions
  Box 3
  12901 Bruce B. Downs Boulevard
  Tampa, FL 33612-4799
  813-974-2229

Emory University
  School of Medicine
  Medical School Admissions, Room 303
  Woodruff Health Sciences Center
  Administration Building
  Atlanta, GA 30322
  404-727-5660

Medical College of Georgia
  School of Medicine
  Associate Dean for Admissions
  Augusta, GA 30912
  404-721-4792

Mercer University
  School of Medicine
  Office of Admissions and Student Affairs
  Macon, GA 31207
  912-752-2524

Morehouse School of Medicine
  Admissions and Student Affairs
  720 Westview Drive, SW
  Atlanta, GA 30310-1495
  404-752-1650

University of Hawaii
  John A. Burns School of Medicine
  Office of Student Affairs
  1960 East-West Road
  Honolulu, HI 96822
  808-948-8300

University of Chicago
  Pritzker School of Medicine
  Office of the Dean of Students
  Billings Hospital, Room G-115A
  5841 South Maryland Avenue, Box 69
  Chicago, IL 60637
  312-702-1939

University of Health Sciences
  Chicago Medical School
  Office of Admissions
  3333 Green Bay Road
  North Chicago, IL 60064
  708-578-3206/3207

University of Illinois
  College of Medicine
  Office of Medical College Admissions
  Room 165 CME M/C 783
  808 South Wood Street
  Chicago, IL 60612
  312-996-5635

Loyola University of Chicago
  Stritch School of Medicine
  Office of Admissions, Room 1752
  2160 South First Avenue
  Maywood, IL 60153
  708-216-3229

Northwestern University Medical School
  Associate Dean for Admissions
  303 East Chicago Avenue
  Chicago, IL 60611
  312-908-8206

Rush Medical College of Rush University
  Office of Admissions
  524 Academic Facility
  600 South Paulina Street
  Chicago, IL 60612
  312-942-6913

Southern Illinois University
  School of Medicine
  Office of Student and Alumni Affairs
  P.O. Box 19230
  Springfield, IL 62794-9230
  217-782-2860

Indiana University
  School of Medicine
  Medical School Admissions Office
  Fesler Hall 213
  1120 South Drive
  Indianapolis, IN 46202-5113
  317-274-3772

University of Iowa
  College of Medicine
  Coordinator of Admissions
  240 Eckstein Medical Research Facility
  Iowa City, IA 52242
  319-335-8052

University of Kansas
  School of Medicine
  Associate Dean for Admissions
  39th and Rainbow Boulevard
  Kansas City, KS 66103

University of Kentucky
    College of Medicine
    Admissions, Room MN-104
    Office of Education
    Chandler Medical Center
    800 Rose Street
    Lexington, KY 40536-0084
    606-233-6161

University of Louisville
    School of Medicine
    Office of Admissions
    Health Sciences Center
    Louisville, KY 40292
    502-588-5193

Louisiana State University
    School of Medicine in New Orleans
    Admissions Office
    1901 Perdido Street
    New Orleans, LA 70112-1393
    504-568-6262

Louisiana State University
    School of Medicine in Shreveport
    Office of Student Admissions
    P.O. Box 33932
    Shreveport, LA 71130-3932
    318-674-5190

Tulane University
    School of Medicine
    Office of Admissions
    1430 Tulane Avenue
    New Orleans, LA 70112
    504-588-5187

Johns Hopkins University
   School of Medicine
   Committee on Admission
   720 Rutland Avenue
   Baltimore, MD 21205-2196
   301-955-3182

University of Maryland
   School of Medicine
   Committee on Admissions
   Room 14-015
   655 West Baltimore Street
   Baltimore, MD 21201
   301-328-7478

Uniformed Services University
     of the Health Sciences
   F. Edward Hebert School of Medicine
   Admissions Office
   Room A-1041
   4301 Jones Bridge Road
   Bethesda, MD 20814-4799
   301-295-3101

Boston University
   School of Medicine
   Admissions Office L-124
   80 East Concord Street
   Boston, MA 02118
   617-638-4633

Harvard Medical School
   Director of Admissions
   25 Shattuck Street
   Boston, MA 02115
   617-432-1550

University of Massachusetts Medical School
    Associate Dean of Admissions
    55 Lake Avenue, North
    Worcester, MA 01655
    508-856-2323

Tufts University
    School of Medicine
    Committee on Admissions
    136 Harrison Avenue
    Boston, MA 02111
    617-956-6571

Michigan State University
    College of Human Medicine
    Office of Admissions
    A-239 Life Sciences
    East Lansing, MI 48824-1317
    517-353-9620

University of Michigan Medical School
    Admissions Office
    M4303 Medical Science Building I
    1301 Catherine Road
    Ann Arbor, MI 48109-0624
    313-764-6317

Wayne State University
    School of Medicine
    Director of Admissions
    540 East Canfield
    Detroit, MI 48201
    313-577-1466

Mayo Medical School
    Admissions Committee
    200 First Street, SW
    Rochester, MN 55905
    507-284-3671

University of Minnesota–Duluth
  School of Medicine
  Office of Admissions, Room 107
  10 University Drive
  Duluth, MN 55812
  218-726-8511

University of Minnesota
  Medical School–Minneapolis
  Office of Admissions and Student Affairs
  Box 293-UMHC
  420 Delaware Street, SE
  Minneapolis, MN 55455-0310
  612-624-1122

University of Mississippi
  School of Medicine
  Chairman, Admissions Committee
  2500 North State Street
  Jackson, MS 39216-4505
  601-984-5010

University of Missouri–Columbia
  School of Medicine
  Office of Admissions
  MA202 Medical Sciences Building
  One Hospital Drive
  Columbia, MO 65212
  314-882-2923

University of Missouri–Kansas City
  School of Medicine
  University Admissions Office
  4825 Troost
  Kansas City, MO 64110
  816-276-1111

Saint Louis University
    School of Medicine
    Ms. Nancy McPeters
    Admissions Committee
    1402 South Grand Boulevard
    St. Louis, MO 63104
    314-577-8205

Washington University
    School of Medicine
    Admissions Office
    660 South Euclid Avenue
    St. Louis, MO 63110
    314-362-6857

Creighton University
    School of Medicine
    Medical School Admissions Office
    California at 24th Street
    Omaha, NE 68178
    402-280-2798

University of Nebraska
    College of Medicine
    Chairman, Admissions Committee
    Room 5017, Wittson Hall
    42nd Street and Dewey Avenue
    Omaha, NE 68105
    402-559-4205

University of Nevada
    School of Medicine
    Office of Admissions
    Reno, NV 89557
    702-784-6001

Dartmouth Medical School
    Office of Admissions
    Hanover, NH 03756
    603-646-7505

University of Medicine and Dentistry of New Jersey
New Jersey Medical School
Director of Admissions
185 South Orange Avenue
Newark, NJ 07103
201-456-4631

University of Medicine and Dentistry of New Jersey
Robert Wood Johnson Medical School
Office of Admissions
675 Hoes Lane
Piscataway, NJ 08854-5635
201-463-4576

University of New Mexico
School of Medicine
Office of Admissions
Basic Medical Sciences Building, Room 107
Albuquerque, NM 87131
505-277-4766

Albany Medical College
Office of Admissions, A-3
47 New Scotland Avenue
Albany, NY 12208
518-445-5521

Albert Einstein College of Medicine of Yeshiva University
Office of Admissions
1300 Morris Park Avenue
Bronx, NY 10461
212-430-2106

Columbia University
College of Physicians and Surgeons
Admissions Office, Room 1-416
630 West 168th Street
New York, NY 10032
212-305-3595

Cornell University Medical College
  Office of Admissions
  445 East 69th Street
  New York, NY 10021
  212-746-1067
Mount Sinai School of Medicine
    of the City University of New York
  Office for Admissions
  Annenberg Building, Room 5-04
  One Gustave L. Levy Place-Box 1002
  New York, NY 10029-6574
  212-241-6696
New York Medical College
  Office of Admissions
  Room 127, Sunshine Cottage
  Valhalla, NY 10595
  914-993-4507
New York University
  School of Medicine
  Office of Admissions
  P.O. Box 1924
  New York, NY 10016
  212-340-5290
University of Rochester
  School of Medicine and Dentistry
  Director of Admissions
  Medical Center Box 601
  Rochester, NY 14642
  716-275-4539
State University of New York
  Health Science Center at Brooklyn
  College of Medicine
  Director of Admissions
  450 Clarkson Avenue—Box 60M
  Brooklyn, NY 11203
  718-270-2737

State University of New York at Buffalo
  School of Medicine and Biomedical Sciences
  Office of Medical Admissions
  Farber Hall, Room 138
  Buffalo, NY 14214
  716-831-3466

State University of New York at Stony Brook
  Health Sciences Center
  School of Medicine
  Committee on Admissions
  Level 4, Room 046
  Stony Brook, NY 11794-8434
  516-444-2113

State University of New York
  Health Science Center at Syracuse
  College of Medicine
  Admissions Committee
  155 Elizabeth Blackwell Street
  Syracuse, NY 13210
  315-464-4570

Bowman Gray School of Medicine of Wake Forest University
  Office of Medical School Admissions
  300 South Hawthorne Road
  Winston-Salem, NC 27103
  919-748-4264

Duke University
  School of Medicine
  Committee on Admissions
  Duke University Medical Center
  P.O. Box 3710
  Durham, NC 27710
  919-684-2985

East Carolina University
   School of Medicine
   Associate Dean
   Office of Admissions
   Greenville, NC 27858-4354
   919-551-2202

University of North Carolina at Chapel Hill
   School of Medicine
   Admissions Office
   CB# 7000 MacNider Hall
   Chapel Hill, NC 27599-7000
   919-962-8331

University of North Dakota
   School of Medicine
   Secretary, Committee on Admissions
   501 Columbia Road
   Grand Forks, ND 58203
   710-777-4221

Case Western Reserve University
   School of Medicine
   Associate Dean for Admissions and Student Affairs
   2119 Abington Road
   Cleveland, OH 44106
   216-368-3450

University of Cincinnati
   College of Medicine
   Office of Admissions
   231 Bethesda Avenue
   Cincinnati, OH 45267-0552
   513-558-7314

Medical College of Ohio
   Admissions Office
   Caller Service No. 10008
   Toledo, OH 43699
   419-381-4229

Northeastern Ohio Universities
   College of Medicine
   Office of Admissions and Educational Research
   P.O. Box 95
   Rootstown, OH 44272
   216-325-2511

Ohio State University
   College of Medicine
   Admissions Committee
   270-A Meiling Hall
   370 West Ninth Avenue
   Columbus, OH 43210-1238
   614-292-7137

Wright State University
   School of Medicine
   Office of Student Affairs/Admissions
   P.O. Box 1751
   Dayton, OH 45401
   513-873-2934

University of Oklahoma
   College of Medicine
   Assistant Director of Student Affairs
   P.O. Box 26901
   Oklahoma City, OK 73190
   405-271-2331

Oregon Health Sciences University
   School of Medicine
   Office of the Registrar, L-109A
   3181 S.W. Sam Jackson Park Road
   Portland, OR 97201
   503-279-7800

Hahnemann University
  School of Medicine
  Medical School Admissions
  Mail Stop 442
  Broad and Vine Streets
  Philadelphia, PA 19102-1192
  215-448-7600

Jefferson Medical College of Thomas Jefferson University
  Associate Dean for Admissions
  1025 Walnut Street
  Philadelphia, PA 19107
  215-928-6983

Medical College of Pennsylvania
  Associate Dean for Student Affairs (Admissions)
  3300 Henry Avenue
  Philadelphia, PA 19129
  215-842-7009

Pennsylvania State University
  College of Medicine
  Office of Student Affairs
  P.O. Box 850
  Hershey, PA 17033
  717-531-8755

University of Pennsylvania
  School of Medicine
  Director of Admissions
  Suite 100–Medical Education Building
  Philadelphia, PA 19104-6056
  215-898-8001

University of Pittsburgh
  School of Medicine
  Office of Admissions
  M-245 Scaife Hall
  Pittsburgh, PA 15261
  412-648-9891

Temple University
   School of Medicine
   Admissions Office
   Suite 305, Student Faculty Center
   Broad and Ontario Streets
   Philadelphia, PA 19140
   215-221-3656

Universidad Central del Caribe
   School of Medicine
   Office of Admissions
   Ramon Ruiz Arnau University Hospital
   Call Box 60-327
   Bayamon, PR 00621-6032
   809-740-4265

Ponce School of Medicine
   Admissions Office
   P.O. Box 7004
   Ponce, PR 00732
   809-840-2575

University of Puerto Rico
   School of Medicine
   Central Admissions Office
   Medical Sciences Campus
   G.P.O. Box 5067
   San Juan, PR 00936
   809-758-2525, Ext. 5213

Brown University
   Program in Medicine
   Office of Admission
   Box G-A212
   Providence, RI 02912
   401-863-2149

Medical University of South Carolina
  College of Medicine
  Director of Admissions
  171 Ashley Avenue
  Charleston, SC 29425
  803-792-3281

University of South Carolina
  School of Medicine
  Senior Associate Dean for Student Programs
  Columbia, SC 29208
  803-733-3325

University of South Dakota
  School of Medicine
  Office of Student Affairs, Room 105
  414 East Clark Street
  Vermillion, SD 57069-2390
  605-677-5233

East Tennessee State University
  James H. Quillen College of Medicine
  Assistant Dean for Admissions and Records
  Quillen-Dishner College of Medicine
  P.O. Box 19,900A
  Johnson City, TN 37614-0002
  615-929-6219

Meharry Medical College
  School of Medicine
  Director, Admissions and Records
  1005 D. B. Todd, Jr. Boulevard
  Nashville, TN 37208
  615-372-6223

University of Tennessee, Memphis
   College of Medicine
   Director of Admissions
   790 Madison Avenue
   Memphis, TN 38163
   901-528-5559

Vanderbilt University
   School of Medicine
   Office of Admissions
   209 Light Hall
   Nashville, TN 37232-0685
   615-322-2145/FAX 343-7286

Baylor College of Medicine
   Office of Admissions
   One Baylor Plaza
   Houston, TX 77030
   713-798-4841

Texas A & M University
   College of Medicine
   Associate Dean for Admissions and Student Affairs
   College Station, TX 77843-1114
   409-845-7744

Texas Tech University
   Health Sciences Center
   School of Medicine
   Office of Admissions
   Lubbock, TX 79430
   806-743-2297

University of Texas
   Southwestern Medical Center at Dallas
   Southwestern Medical School
   Office of the Registrar
   5323 Harry Hines Boulevard
   Dallas, TX 75235-9096
   214-688-2670

University of Texas
  Medical School at Galveston
  Office of Admissions
  G.210, Ashbel Smith Building, Rt. M-17
  Galveston, TX 77550
  409-761-3517

University of Texas
  Medical School at Houston
  Office of Admissions-Room G-024
  P.O. Box 20708
  Houston, TX 77225
  713-792-4711

University of Texas
  Medical School at San Antonio
  Registrar's Office
  7703 Floyd Curl Drive
  San Antonio, TX 78284-7701
  512-567-2665

University of Utah
  School of Medicine
  Director, Medical School Admissions
  50 North Medical Drive
  Salt Lake City, UT 84132
  801-581-7498

University of Vermont
  College of Medicine
  Admissions Office
  E-109 Given Building
  Burlington, VT 05405
  802-656-2154

Eastern Virginia Medical School of the Medical College of
   Hampton Roads
   Office of Admissions
   700 Olney Road
   Norfolk, VA 23507
   804-446-5812

Virginia Commonwealth University
   Medical College of Virginia
   School of Medicine
   Medical School Admissions
   MCV Station, Box 565
   Richmond, VA 23298-0565
   804-786-9630

University of Virginia
   School of Medicine
   Medical School Admissions Office
   Box 235
   Charlottesville, VA 22908
   804-924-5571

University of Washington
   School of Medicine
   Admissions Office (SM-22)
   Health Sciences Center T-545
   Seattle, WA 98195
   206-543-7212

Marshall University
   School of Medicine
   Admissions Office
   1542 Spring Valley Drive
   Huntington, WV 25755
   304-696-7312; 800-544-8514

West Virginia University
  School of Medicine
  Office of Admissions and Records
  Health Sciences Center
  Morgantown, WV 26506
  304-293-3521

Medical College of Wisconsin
  Office of Admissions and Registrar
  8701 Watertown Plank Road
  Milwaukee, WI 53226
  414-257-8246

University of Wisconsin Medical School
  Admissions Committee
  Medical Sciences Center, Room 1205
  1300 University Avenue
  Madison, WI 53706
  608-263-4925

GEOGRAPHICAL LISTING OF MEDICAL SCHOOLS

Alabama
University of Alabama School of Medicine
University of South Alabama College of Medicine
Arizona
University of Arizona College of Medicine
Arkansas
University of Arkansas College of Medicine
California
University of California, Davis, School of Medicine
University of California, Irvine, College of Medicine
University of California, Los Angeles, UCLA School of Medicine
University of California, San Diego, School of Medicine
University of California, San Francisco, School of Medicine
Loma Linda University School of Medicine
University of Southern California School of Medicine
Stanford University School of Medicine
Colorado
University of Colorado School of Medicine
Connecticut
University of Connecticut School of Medicine
Yale University School of Medicine
District of Columbia
George Washington University School of Medicine and Health Sciences
Georgetown University School of Medicine
Howard University College of Medicine

Florida
University of Florida College of Medicine
University of Miami School of Medicine
University of South Florida College of Medicine
Georgia
Emory University School of Medicine
Medical College of Georgia School of Medicine
Mercer University School of Medicine
Morehouse School of Medicine
Hawaii
University of Hawaii John A. Burns School of Medicine
Illinois
University of Chicago Pritzker School of Medicine
University of Health Sciences/Chicago Medical School
University of Illinois College of Medicine
Loyola University of Chicago Stritch School of Medicine
Northwestern University Medical School
Rush Medical College of Rush University
Southern Illinois University School of Medicine
Indiana
Indiana University School of Medicine
Iowa
University of Iowa College of Medicine
Kansas
University of Kansas School of Medicine
Kentucky
University of Kentucky College of Medicine
University of Louisville School of Medicine
Louisiana
Louisiana State University School of Medicine in New Orleans
Louisiana State University School of Medicine in Shreveport
Tulane University School of Medicine
Maryland
Johns Hopkins University School of Medicine
University of Maryland School of Medicine
Uniformed Services University of the Health Sciences—F. Edward
  Hebert School of Medicine
Massachusetts
Boston University School of Medicine
Harvard Medical School

University of Massachusetts Medical School
Tufts University School of Medicine
Michigan
Michigan State University College of Human Medicine
University of Michigan Medical School
Wayne State University School of Medicine
Minnesota
Mayo Medical School
University of Minnesota—Duluth School of Medicine
University of Minnesota Medical School—Minneapolis
Mississippi
University of Mississippi School of Medicine
Missouri
University of Missouri—Columbia School of Medicine
University of Missouri—Kansas City School of Medicine
Saint Louis University School of Medicine
Washington University School of Medicine
Nebraska
Creighton University School of Medicine
University of Nebraska College of Medicine
Nevada
University of Nevada School of Medicine
New Hampshire
Dartmouth Medical School
New Jersey
University of Medicine and Dentistry of New Jersey—New Jersey
  Medical School
University of Medicine and Dentistry of New Jersey—Robert Wood
  Johnson Medical School
New Mexico
University of New Mexico School of Medicine
New York
Albany Medical College
Albert Einstein College of Medicine of Yeshiva University
Columbia University College of Physicians and Surgeons
Cornell University Medical College
Mount Sinai School of Medicine of the City University of New York
New York Medical College
New York University School of Medicine
University of Rochester School of Medicine and Dentistry

State University of New York Health Science Center at Brooklyn
College of Medicine
State University of New York at Buffalo School of Medicine and
Biomedical Sciences
State University of New York at Stony Brook Health Sciences Center
School of Medicine
State University of New York Health Science Center at Syracuse
College of Medicine
North Carolina
Bowman Gray School of Medicine of Wake Forest University
Duke University School of Medicine
East Carolina University School of Medicine
University of North Carolina at Chapel Hill School of Medicine
North Dakota
University of North Dakota School of Medicine
Ohio
Case Western Reserve University School of Medicine
University of Cincinnati College of Medicine
Medical College of Ohio
Northeastern Ohio Universities College of Medicine
Ohio State University College of Medicine
Wright State University School of Medicine
Oklahoma
University of Oklahoma College of Medicine
Oregon
Oregon Health Sciences University School of Medicine
Pennsylvania
Hahnemann University School of Medicine
Jefferson Medical College of Thomas Jefferson University
Medical College of Pennsylvania
Pennsylvania State University College of Medicine
University of Pennsylvania School of Medicine
University of Pittsburgh School of Medicine
Temple University School of Medicine
Puerto Rico
Universidad Central del Caribe School of Medicine
Ponce School of Medicine
University of Puerto Rico School of Medicine
Rhode Island
Brown University Program in Medicine

South Carolina
Medical University of South Carolina College of Medicine
University of South Carolina School of Medicine
South Dakota
University of South Dakota School of Medicine
Tennessee
East Tennessee State University Quillen-Dishner College of Medicine
Meharry Medical College School of Medicine
University of Tennessee, Memphis, College of Medicine
Vanderbilt University School of Medicine
Texas
Baylor College of Medicine
Texas A & M University College of Medicine
Texas Tech University Health Sciences Center School of Medicine
University of Texas Southwestern Medical Center at Dallas
    Southwestern Medical School
University of Texas Medical School at Galveston
University of Texas Medical School at Houston
University of Texas Medical School at San Antonio
Utah
University of Utah School of Medicine
Vermont
University of Vermont College of Medicine
Virginia
Eastern Virginia Medical School of the Medical College of Hampton
    Roads
Virginia Commonwealth University Medical College of Virginia
    School of Medicine
University of Virginia School of Medicine
Washington
University of Washington School of Medicine
West Virginia
Marshall University School of Medicine
West Virginia University School of Medicine
Wisconsin
Medical College of Wisconsin
University of Wisconsin Medical School

APPENDIX D

COMBINED DEGREE PROGRAMS

The following is a list of the programs that combine the baccalaureate degree with an M.D. degree. In some cases, these programs may be completed in less than eight years.

University of California, Riverside and
University of California, Los Angeles,
*   UCLA School of Medicine*

This program offers an accelerated curriculum which allows receipt of a B.S. degree after four years of college work and the M.D. degree seven years after matriculation as an undergraduate freshman.

Student Affairs Officer
  Division of Biomedical Sciences
  University of California, Riverside
  Riverside, CA 92521-0121
  714-787-4333

Howard University

The aims of this combined-degree program are to encourage bright young students to choose medicine as a career and to enter Howard University College of Medicine for their medical education. Curriculum can be completed in seven years.

Director
  Center for Preprofessional Education
  P.O. Box 1124
  Administration Building
  Howard University
  Washington, DC 20059
  202-636-6200

University of Miami

The Honors Program in Engineering and Medicine trains physicians who can understand, utilize, and further advance biomedical engineering technologies in their areas of specialization. The curriculum can take either six or seven years to complete.

Office of Admissions
  P.O. Box 24805
  Coral Gables, FL 33124
  305-284-4323

Northwestern University

The honors program in medical education provides students with an individualized undergraduate curriculum that shortens the premedical preparation and assures entry to medical school. The curriculum normally takes seven years.

Office of Admission and Financial Aid
  1801 Hinman Avenue
  Evanston, IL 60204-3060
  708-491-7271

Louisiana State University
School of Medicine in Shreveport

This combined-degree program provides outstanding high school seniors with an opportunity to complete the prerequisite undergraduate preparation and medical school in six years.

Office of Student Admissions
  P.O. Box 33932
  Shreveport, LA 71130-3932

Boston University

The combined-degree program provides an undergraduate premedical preparation that emphasizes the humanities and social sciences, and affords a quality medical education even though the overall period of study is shortened. The program takes seven years with a six- or eight-year option.

Associate Director, Admissions
  121 Bay State Road
  Boston, MA 02215
  617-353-2333

University of Michigan

The primary goal of the Integrated Premedical/Medical (Inteflex) Program is to educate physicians who are scientifically competent, compassionate, and socially conscious and who can apply the insights gained in the study of the humanities and social sciences to the problems of medical practice. The curriculum normally takes seven years to complete.

Inteflex Program
  2715 Furstenberg
  Ann Arbor, MI 48109-0611
  313-764-9534

University of Missouri–Kansas City
School of Medicine

This combined baccalaureate-M.D. degree program integrates the humanities, basic sciences, and clinical medicine throughout the curriculum so graduates will have the background for lifelong learning in order to meet the needs of their patients. The curriculum normally takes six years to complete.

Council on Selection
  2411 Holmes
  Kansas City, MO 64108
  816-235-1900

Washington University School of Medicine

The Scholars Program in Medicine provides an eight-year program which should produce future leaders in American medicine. Entrants to the undergraduate phase of the program are given a provisional acceptance to Washington University School of Medicine and encouraged to concentrate on learning and scholarship by exploring broad areas of interest during their undergraduate years.

Coordinator, Scholars Program in Medicine
  Campus Box 1089
  One Brookings Drive
  St. Louis, MO 63130
  314-889-6000

Rutgers University and
University of Medicine and Dentistry of New Jersey—
  Robert Wood Johnson Medical School

The program permits the early identification and admission of high-quality medical students. It also integrates medical studies with liberal arts study. The program is eight years in duration.

Bachelor/Medical Degree Program
  Nelson Biological Laboratory
  P.O. Box 1059
  Piscataway, NJ 08855-1059
  201-932-5270

Brooklyn College and
State University of New York
  Health Science Center at Brooklyn
  College of Medicine

The aims of this program are to produce physicians who are humanists and to offer an economically sound path to medicine. The program is seven years in length with an eight-year option.

Director of Admissions
1203 James Hall
Brooklyn, NY 11210
718-780-5044

New York University

The goal of the B.A./M.D. program is to train broadly educated doctors who are interested in people and their place in society and who are excited about the science of medicine. The program is eight years in length.

Graham R. Underwood, Ph.D.
  Director, B.A./M.D. Program
  New York University
  College of Arts and Science
  100 Washington Square East
  Main Building, Room 904
  New York, NY 10003
  212-998-8160

*Rensselaer Polytechnic Institute
and Albany Medical College*

The six-year biomedical program offers qualified individuals the opportunity to earn the B.S. and M.D. degrees in six calendar years. Participants receive a strong science-based education in a technological university before entering Albany Medical College.

Admissions Counselor
  Troy, NY 12180
  518-276-6216

*Sophie Davis School of Biomedical Education—
  City University of New York*

The purposes of this combined-degree program are to train primary care physicians who will work in medically underserved urban areas and to increase the number of minority physicians. This seven-year program leads to a baccalaureate degree granted by the City College of New York and to the M.D. degree awarded by one of eight New York medical schools.

Office of Admissions
  138th Street and Convent Avenue
  New York, NY 10031
  212-690-8256

State University of New York at Stony Brook

The purpose of this program is to provide for early selection of students for medical school. It does not take an accelerated approach to medical education.

Faculty Associate for Health Professions
Office of Undergraduate Studies
Library E3320
Stony Brook, NY 11794-3351
516-632-7032

Union College and
Albany Medical College

Stressing both the sciences and humanities, the seven-year program in medical education offers students the opportunity to earn the B.S. degree and the M.D. degree in seven years.

Associate Dean of Admissions
Schenectady, NY 12308
518-370-6591

Case Western Reserve University

This program is intended to provide college students with a greater sense of freedom and choice in the pursuit of a premedical baccalaureate degree. This program takes eight years to complete.

Office of Undergraduate Admission
Tomlinson Hall
10900 Euclid Avenue
Cleveland, OH 44106-4901
216-368-4450

Northeastern Ohio Universities
  College of Medicine

The purpose of this college of medicine is to prepare well-trained medical doctors who can enter any field of practice, particularly at the community level. This is one of the few United States medical schools which exclusively offers a combined-degree program to its students. For 60 percent of the students admitted, the curriculum takes six years to complete and for the remainder, seven years.

Admissions Office
  P. O. Box 44272
  1-800-686-2511 (in Ohio)
  216-325-2511 (outside Ohio)

Gannon University
and Hahnemann University
  School of Medicine

The Cooperative Program for Education of Physicians in Pennsylvania emphasizes, but is not limited to, the preparation of family physicians. This seven-year program leads to a baccalaureate degree from Gannon University and to the M.D. degree from Hahnemann University School of Medicine.

Gannon-Hahnemann 7-Year B.S./M.D. Program
  Office of Admissions
  University Square
  Erie, PA 16541
  814-871-7407

*Lehigh University
and Medical College of Pennsylvania*

This program gives gifted high school students who are certain that they want to become physicians the opportunity to obtain a diversified education and to reduce their total education cost. This program, normally six years in duration, allows students to obtain a bachelor's degree from Lehigh University and an M.D. degree from the Medical College of Pennsylvania.

Office of Admissions
  Alumni Building 27
  Bethlehem, PA 18105
  215-758-3100

*Pennsylvania State University
and Jefferson Medical College
  of Thomas Jefferson University*

This program, which began in 1963, is a cooperative effort between Pennsylvania State University and Jefferson Medical College of Thomas Jefferson University in Philadelphia. Students can earn both the B.S. and M.D. degrees in six calendar years after graduation from high school.

Undergraduate Admissions Office
  201 Shields Building
  Box 3000
  University Park, PA 16802
  814-865-5479

Brown University

The Program in Liberal Medical Education combines liberal arts and professional education to enable each student to develop graduate level competence in a chosen field of scholarship. Great flexibility is built into the program. Each student develops an individualized educational plan in close collaboration with faculty advisors. The program takes eight years to complete.

Coordinator
Program in Liberal Medical Education
Box G
Providence, RI 02912
401-863-2450

University of Wisconsin-Madison Medical School

The Medical Scholars Program provides conditional admission to the University of Wisconsin-Madison Medical School for 50 highly qualified Wisconsin high school seniors. Medical scholars are a part of the medical school community and may participate in specially designed basic science and clinical experiences. The program takes seven to nine years to complete.

Medical Scholars Program
1300 University Avenue, Room 1205
Madison, WI 53706
608-263-4920

*University of Wisconsin-Milwaukee
and Medical College of Wisconsin*

The Target M.D. Program provides a well-rounded pre-medical curriculum together with a rigorous four-year medical education to a group of carefully selected students who will benefit from an accelerated program. This is a seven-year program.

Target M.D. Program
  College of Letters and Science
  P.O. Box 413
  Milwaukee, WI 53201
  414-229-6104

SPECIALTY BOARDS

Allergy and Immunology

American Board of Allergy and Immunology
    University City Science Center
    3624 Market Street
    Philadelphia, PA 19104

Anesthesiology

American Board of Anesthesiology
    100 Constitution Plaza
    Hartford, CT 06103

Colon and Rectal Surgery

American Board of Colon and Rectal Surgery
    8750 Telegraph, Suite 410
    Taylor, MI 48180

Dermatology

American Board of Dermatology
Henry Ford Hospital
Detroit, MI 48202

Emergency Medicine

American Board of Emergency Medicine
200 Woodland Pass, Suite D
East Lansing, MI 48823

Family Practice

American Board of Family Practice
2228 Young Drive
Lexington, KY 40505

Internal Medicine

American Board of Internal Medicine
University City Science Center
3624 Market Street
Philadelphia, PA 19104

Neurological Surgery

American Board of Neurological Surgery
P.O. Box 4056
Chapel Hill, NC 27515-4056

Nuclear Medicine

American Board of Nuclear Medicine
900 Veteran Avenue, Room 12-200
Los Angeles, CA 90024

Obstetrics & Gynecology

American Board of Obstetrics and Gynecology
4225 Roosevelt Way, NE, Suite 305
Seattle, WA 98105

Ophthalmology

American Board of Ophthalmology
111 Presidential Boulevard, Suite 241
Bala Cynwyd, PA 19004

Orthopedic Surgery

American Board of Orthopaedic Surgery
737 North Michigan Avenue, Suite 1150
Chicago, IL 60611

Otolaryngology

American Board of Otolaryngology
5615 Kirby Drive, Suite 936
Houston, TX 77005

Pathology

American Board of Pathology
5401 West Kennedy Boulevard
P.O. Box 25915
Tampa, FL 33622

Pediatrics

American Board of Pediatrics
111 Silver Cedar Court
Chapel Hill, NC 27514

Physical Medicine and Rehabilitation

American Board of Physical Medicine and Rehabilitation
    Suite 674, Norwest Center
    21 First Street, SW
    Rochester, MN 55902

Plastic Surgery

American Board of Plastic Surgery
    1617 John F. Kennedy Boulevard, #860
    Philadelphia, PA 19103

Preventive Medicine

American Board of Preventive Medicine
    Department of Community Medicine
    Wright State University School of Medicine
    P.O. Box 927
    Dayton, OH 45401

Psychiatry and Neurology

American Board of Psychiatry and Neurology
    500 Lake Cook Road, #335
    Deerfield, IL 60015

Radiology

American Board of Radiology
    300 Park, Suite 440
    Birmingham, MI 48009

Surgery

American Board of Surgery
   1617 John F. Kennedy Boulevard, Suite 860
   Philadelphia, PA 19103-1847

Thoracic Surgery

American Board of Thoracic Surgery
   One Rotary Center, Suite 803
   Evanston, IL 60201

Urology

American Board of Urology
   31700 Telegraph Road, Suite 150
   Birmingham, MI 48010

A complete list of titles in our extensive *Opportunities* series

OPPORTUNITIES IN
Accounting
Acting
Advertising
Aerospace
Airline
Animal & Pet Care
Architecture
Automotive Service
Banking
Beauty Culture
Biological Sciences
Biotechnology
Broadcasting
Building Construction Trades
Business Communication
Business Management
Cable Television
CAD/CAM
Carpentry
Chemistry
Child Care
Chiropractic
Civil Engineering
Cleaning Service
Commercial Art & Graphic
  Design
Computer Maintenance
Computer Science
Counseling & Development
Crafts
Culinary
Customer Service
Data Processing
Dental Care
Desktop Publishing
Direct Marketing
Drafting
Electrical Trades
Electronics
Energy
Engineering
Engineering Technology
Environmental
Eye Care
Farming and Agriculture
Fashion
Fast Food
Federal Government
Film
Financial

Fire Protection Services
Fitness
Food Services
Foreign Language
Forestry
Franchising
Gerontology & Aging Services
Health & Medical
Heating, Ventilation, Air
  Conditioning, and
  Refrigeration
High Tech
Home Economics
Homecare Services
Horticulture
Hospital Administration
Hotel & Motel Management
Human Resource Management
Information Systems
Installation & Repair
Insurance
Interior Design & Decorating
International Business
Journalism
Laser Technology
Law
Law Enforcement & Criminal
  Justice
Library & Information Science
Machine Trades
Marine & Maritime
Marketing
Masonry
Medical Imaging
Medical Technology
Mental Health
Metalworking
Military
Modeling
Music
Nonprofit Organizations
Nursing
Nutrition
Occupational Therapy
Office Occupations
Paralegal
Paramedical
Part-time & Summer Jobs
Performing Arts
Petroleum
Pharmacy
Photography

Physical Therapy
Physician
Physician Assistant
Plastics
Plumbing & Pipe Fitting
Postal Service
Printing
Property Management
Psychology
Public Health
Public Relations
Publishing
Purchasing
Real Estate
Recreation & Leisure
Religious Service
Restaurant
Retailing
Robotics
Sales
Secretarial
Social Science
Social Work
Special Education
Speech-Language Patholo
Sports & Athletics
Sports Medicine
State & Local Governmen
Teaching
Teaching English to Speak
  of Other Languages
Technical Writing &
  Communications
Telecommunications
Telemarketing
Television & Video
Theatrical Design &
  Production
Tool & Die
Transportation
Travel
Trucking
Veterinary Medicine
Visual Arts
Vocational & Technical
Warehousing
Waste Management
Welding
Word Processing
Writing
Your Own Service Busines

VGM Career Horizons
a division of *NTC Publishing Group*
4255 West Touhy Avenue
Lincolnwood, Illinois 60646–1975